The Magic Makeover

The Magic Makeover

Tricks for Looking Thinner, Younger, and More Confident—

Instantly!

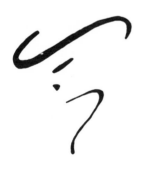

by *LYNDA MILLNER*

EDITED BY CORK MILLNER
DRAWINGS BY ANDREA

Fithian Press
Santa Barbara, 1997

SECOND PRINTING

Published by Fithian Press
A division of Daniel and Daniel, Publishers, Inc.
Post Office Box 1525
Santa Barbara, CA 93102

Book design: Eric Larson
CATHY™ cartoon strips reprinted with permission of Guisewite Studio

LIBRARY OF CONGRESS CATALOGING-IN-PUBLICATION DATA
Millner, Lynda.
    The magic makeover : tricks for looking thinner, younger, and more confident—
instantly! / by Lynda Millner ; edited by Cork Millner ; illustrated by Andrea.
        p. cm.
        ISBN 1-56474-222-9 (pbk.)
        1. Beauty, Personal.   I. Millner, Cork, (date).   II. Title.
RA778.M634   1997
646.7'024—dc21   97-3655
                                                               CIP

Contents

To Cork

Without whom this book never would have happened.
You really are the "wind beneath my wings."

Beauty is eternity gazing at
itself in the mirror
But you are that eternity and you
are that mirror

—*Kahlil Gibran, The Prophet*

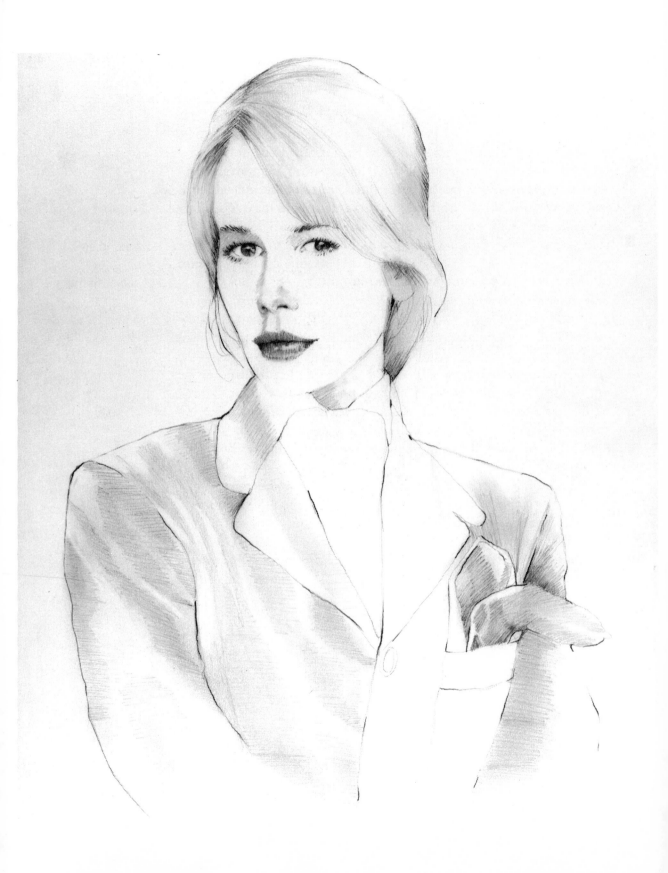

CHAPTER ONE

The Instant Magic Makeover

Magic Tricks to Go from So-So to So Stunning

*"The reason I don't have a handgun in
the house is I would have shot off
my thighs years ago."*

—Oprah Winfrey

Let's face it, you're less than perfect.

Like me.

The average American woman is 5'4" tall, weighs 143 pounds, and wears a size 12 to 14.

The average fashion model is 5'10" tall, weighs little enough to classify as anorexic, and wears a size 6 to 8. Models (and most actresses and dancers) are thinner than 95 percent of the women out there.

Take that as a compliment. That makes you "normal."

Unfortunately, all you see in fashion magazines, on television, and on the movie theater screen are beautiful, skinny, *perfect* women. No wonder we are obsessed with being thin and trying to be perfect. You'd look glamorous too if you had a makeup artist fussing over every pore, a hairstylist fiddling with every strand of hair, and a fashion designer fidgeting with the drapery of your dress.

Sometimes when I am at a social function I pretend in

my mind to be a fairy godmother with the ability to wave my wand over women who dress completely wrong for their figure, color, lifestyle, and image. In the stardust from the wand I completely make them over, and they materialize well-dressed and properly made up. I create a princess. Unfortunately the clock chimes twelve, and the woman has not changed. But if I had the time to spend with that person (and she were willing to listen) I could make her over.

Did you ever watch those "makeovers" on the Oprah Winfrey Show? Oprah and her staff select a woman from the audience who looks like she dressed in the dark—baggy tee shirt with a motto that says "Physically Pfhittt," sweat pants, grungy tennis shoes—and then they have a hairstylist, makeup artist, and fashion expert transform her "instantly" into one of those perfect people. The audience ohhs and ahhs, the woman's husband (who looks like he's dressed for a beer-guzzling contest) is in shock, and the woman glows under the spotlight. Of course, like Cinderella's carriage turning back into a pumpkin, the woman will revert to "Physically Pfhittt" the next morning. Yet, for that one magical moment, that woman, that size-14 woman, that woman who had no sense of style or image, looked great!

And so can you.

With the proper clothes you can fake out fat, belittle your behind, and whittle away a not-so-little middle. With the proper makeup and hairstyle you will be off to a great adventure with a wonderful scenic view at the end—a new you:

Thinner
Younger
More confident
Instantly!

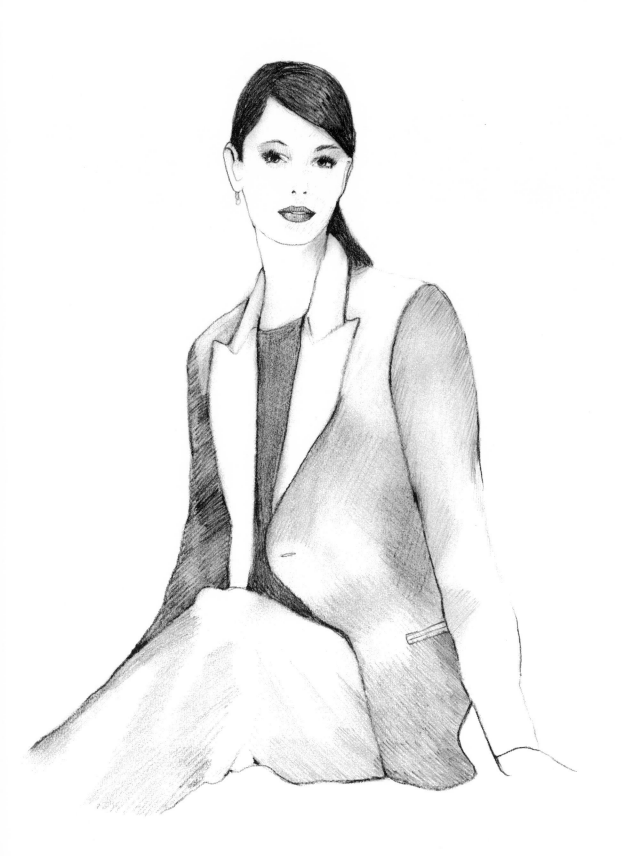

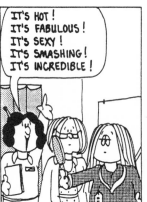
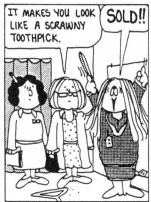
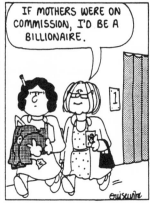

THINNING MAGIC TRICKS

Restyling Barbara Bush

If I could choose one woman in the U.S. to make over instantly, I'd choose Barbara Bush (a sweet, charming lady whom I admire). But…she's famous for the choker of pearls that she wears to hide neck wrinkles. The choker makes her large frame and thick neck look even thicker. If she'd wear long ropes of pearls, she'd look thinner—instantly.

Mrs. Bush also loves print dresses and suits with pleated skirts—both of which tend to make her look like a sofa instead of the regal lady she is. I would never have her wear double-breasted outfits of any kind; always single-breasted with just a hint of fitting at the waist to give her more shape.

These tips for the ex-first lady would not compromise the unique "style" that she's developed through the years; they would only enhance that style—and slim her body.

You too can look thinner by following these ten instant steps.

TEN INSTANT STEPS TO LOOKING THINNER

1. **Shoulder Pads** If you have narrow shoulders and wide hips (eggplant shape) always use shoulder pads in blouses and jackets.

2. **Color Column** One stroke of color from shoulder to shoes makes you appear taller and thinner. Wear dark or monochromatic colors.

3. **Horizontal vs. Vertical Stripes** This is an old tactic to give the illusion of slimness, but you still see overweight women wearing broad horizontal stripes.

4. **Push Up Sleeves** This is an optical illusion that makes partially bare arms appear slimmer than ones in long sleeves. It shaves off five pounds from your silhouette.

5. **Jacket Length** Longer jackets that cover your hips and bottom fade away pounds.

6. **Skirt Length** Never let the hemline of your skirt end at the heaviest part of your leg.

7. **Pants** The narrower the pants, the wider the hips. Straight or wider pant legs narrow the hips.

8. **Belts** Drape a chain belt around your waist. Diagonal lines slim.

9. **Choker Necklaces** Chokers (as we noted with Barbara Bush) can make you shorter and wider. Long necklaces lengthen and narrow your face, neck, and body.

10. **Strappy Shoes** Shoes with straps will make your legs look larger. A pump will slim them, especially ones with a low vamp.

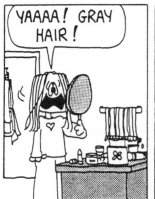 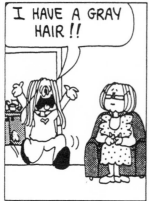 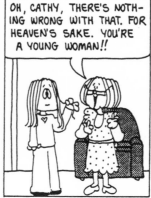 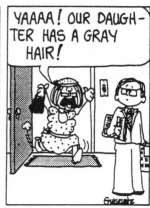

YOUTHFUL MAGIC TRICKS

Flossie Smedly-Headly—Aging By Denial

The society doyenne—let's call her Flossie Smedly-Headly—is aging by denial. Her jet-black hair has gray roots, her cupid's bow mouth (in garish red lipstick) is right out of silent films, and her fussy clothes make her look like she's going to the homecoming prom. She wears too many jewels to charity bashes—a Tiffany display counter's worth of them. Flossie proves the fact that money doesn't make you well dressed. Underneath that clown's mask of makeup and plastic hair is a woman of sixty trying to look like she did in college. It just doesn't work.

But you can appear younger than you are and be more vibrant by following these ten instant steps.

TEN INSTANT STEPS TO LOOKING YOUNGER

1. **Flattering Colors** Wear colors that flatter your skin tone. Your wrinkles will be less distinct, your skin a more youthful color. Even your teeth look whiter, your eyes brighter. It's like getting an instant face lift.

2. **For Younger Eyes** Absolutely no frosted shadows or blush if you have crepey lids. It's like advertising your age lines.

3. **Curling Eyelashes** Use an eyelash curler for an instant eye lift.

4. **Wear Contemporary Makeup** Throw away that orange lip gloss and that blue eye shadow that you have loved for the last fifteen years.

5. **Hair Color** If you were a brunette, your natural silver color should be striking. If allowing your hair to gray is not your thing, be sure to avoid a brassy mane of blond locks or a *very dark* color. Those will only make your wrinkles show more. Try highlighting, reverse streaking, or soft color.

6. **Get a Contemporary Hairstyle** Maturity doesn't *demand* short "helmet head" hair. Take off years with an up-to-date hairstyle, one created especially for your face, neck, and body.

7. **Be in Style** Wear clothes that show you're a woman of today—not ten-year-old "classics." Don't always wear pants; try a skirt. It will make you feel and look younger.

8. **Revitalize Your Skirt Length** Mid-calf lengths look dowdy. Wear skirts above the knee, just below the knee, boot length, or all the way to the floor.

9. **Grandma Shoes** Don't wear matronly shoes. There are lots of smart, comfortable styles available.

10. **Change Your Attitude** Age is an attitude. Be sure your attitude is young. Be flexible. Rigidity spells A-G-E.

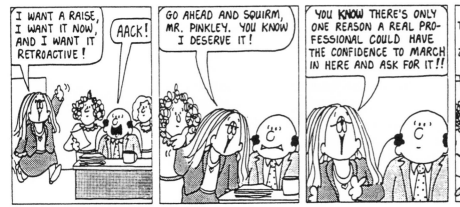
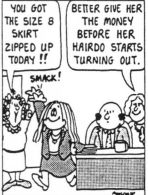

CONFIDENCE MAGIC TRICKS

Sophia Loren's Aura of Self-Confidence

Sophia Loren admits that as a young girl she was known as "Toothpick." She once said, "I was thin as a beanpole, tumbling over myself like a newborn colt." When she began her movie career as a teenager, she was so tall and awkward she was nicknamed "Giraffe." After an early screen test, Loren was told there was no way the camera could make her look good. She was also asked to have her nose "trimmed off a bit."

But the girl within didn't see what the camera or the mirror saw. In her book, *Women & Beauty*, Loren wrote, "A journalist once said of me that my mouth was too large, my nose too long, my chin and lips too broad, and yet the sum of my parts is somehow beautiful." Although she did not consider herself beautiful, she was aware of her allure. She decided to learn how to create illusions to enhance her face and figure, and she had the *confidence* to make the changes.

You too can appear confident by following these ten steps.

TEN INSTANT STEPS TO BEING CONFIDENT

1. **The Fig Leaf** Clasping your hands together in front of you like a fig leaf tells everyone that, at that moment, you are uncomfortable and don't know what to do with your hands. Let them hang (or place them in your pockets).

2. **Walk Tall** Stand up straight! Don't slump, even if you are very tall. Good posture makes people feel you have something to say.

3. **A Firm Handshake** Don't offer a "dead fish" handshake. Grasp the hand of everyone you meet *firmly.* Offer your full hand, not just the fingers.

4. **Maintain Eye Contact** Dropping your eyes or staring at someone's earlobe means you're not comfortable. Having eye-to-eye contact means you have self-esteem.

5. **The Confident Walk** Head up, eyes forward, arms swinging naturally at your sides, a pleasant I'm-all-here look on your face.

6. **Sit Like a Queen** When you sit, anchor one foot on the floor and tuck the other foot behind it at the ankle. It looks elegant and will keep you from fidgeting.

7. **Wear a Hat** Hats attract attention. When you wear a hat people assume you are confident. You will even get better service.

8. **Get in Style** Putting on the right makeup, having the right hairstyle, and wearing the right colors not only make you look like a million, but give you the aura that "this lady has it all together."

9. **Forget the Flaws** If you don't like your nose, abhor your toes, think your ears look like Dumbo's, then *don't tell anyone.* Never broadcast what you perceive to be your flaws. If you don't point them out, the odds are no one will notice.

10. **Be Positive** A positive attitude makes people want to be with you because you project an aura of confidence.

Now it is time to reach deep into our magician's hat—and pull out the *The Magic Makeover*.

The Magic Makeover will show you how a little creative abracadabra can give the illusion of looking wonderful with a less-than-perfect body. Like a magician, you can maximize your best parts and minimize your bad parts. You can go from so-so to so stunning—instantly.

Let the magic begin!

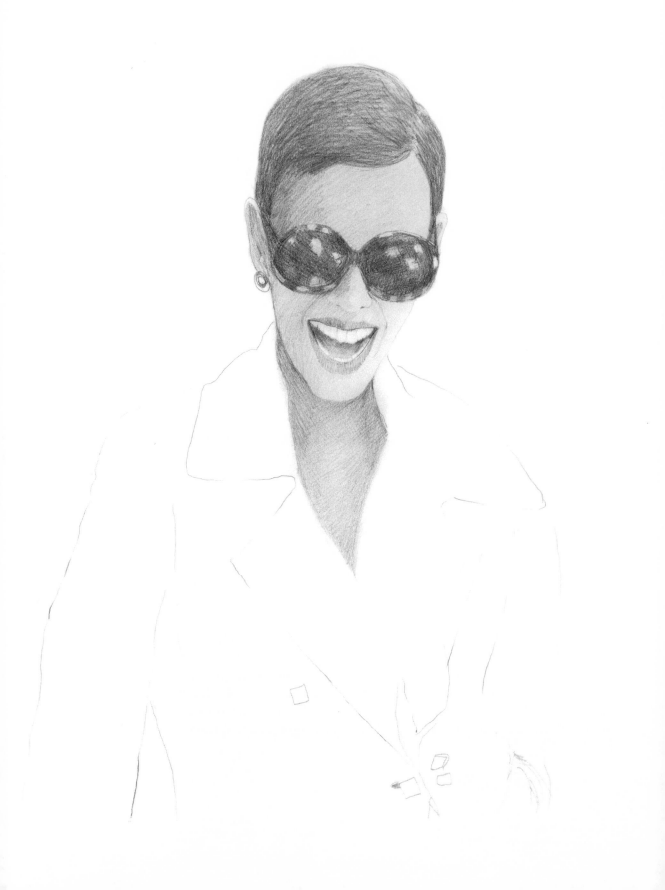

CHAPTER TWO

Image Management

How to Analyze Your Image

*"People are like stained-glass windows.
They sparkle like crystal in the sun, but
when darkness comes, they continue to
shine only if there's a light from within."*

—Anonymous

W here did those two weird-looking people come from?" The whispered comment was faint behind me.

Then came the hushed answer: *"She looks awful."*

I knew I looked awful. I had *purposely* dressed to look awful. And I had a horrible headache.

I caught a glimpse of myself in the wall-size mirror that hung on one side of the crowded formal banquet room. Ugh! I might as well be in sneakers, cutoffs, and a sweatshirt that said "Not a Well Woman." I was a walking rhetoric of unfashionable excess; I had pinned on a long hairpiece that spread over my shoulders, exaggerating my already long face, and added outdated false eyelashes and 1970s makeup that made me look washed out. My miniskirt was out of style, the sweater too tight, and the pantyhose too pale for my legs. As an added abuse I had on a pair of unflattering shoes.

I looked tacky.

My husband beside me was no better off in pants that were too short, a baggy tweed jacket, dark shirt, and string tie.

We were a mess.

I turned from the mirror as the fashionably attired hostess reluctantly introduced my husband and me to a prominent city attorney. The hostess said something about "the hors d'oeuvres…" and vanished. My husband offered the attorney a limp handshake, and I smiled thinly. I felt like I had a piece of spinach stuck between my teeth. The attorney hastily excused himself and left, totally turned off.

Ninety-five percent

The director of the model agency where my husband and I worked as fashion models walked up. She was, as usual, elegantly *of our first impression* coifed and gowned. She grinned at her two guinea pigs and said *is non-verbal.* with a secret smile, "You're both doing great."

"I feel like a fool," I said, forcing a smile. This wasn't the real me. Even as a little girl, I could never dress up for a costume party as a clown or wear funny faces. I had to be the princess. "I can feel the people rejecting us because of the way we look," I whispered to the director.

"See, it's working."

"And my headache is getting worse."

"Your husband seems to be enjoying himself."

"He's an exhibitionist."

She patted me on the shoulder maternally. "Don't worry, it won't be long. Right after dinner I'll give my talk on style and image, then…" she leaned in "…then I'll unveil you."

I sighed.

"Come on, I'll introduce you to my husband," she said.

"Have you told him?" I asked hopefully.

"No. Not one of these gorgeous people knows." She smiled real big. "Isn't this fun?"

When the agency director first approached my husband and me with the idea of being a couple of macabre mannequins, it had sounded like fun. Just come to a large fancy banquet poorly dressed, and let her remake us in front of the audience. *"Voila!"* she had said. "Instant image improvement."

It was a *long* dinner. I sat opposite her husband, who spent all his time talking to his tablemate—the attorney.

My head was pounding.

Finally, the director was introduced and got up to do her presentation. She asked for two volunteers from the audience, people whose "images" she could "reconstruct."

I quickly raised my hand, as did my husband.

Everyone breathed a sigh of relief. We were obviously in deep need of heavy reconstruction.

We stood in front of the guests on a small stage near the lectern, and the agency director helped us with our posture and showed us how to walk. She then studied us closely and said, "I really need to help you with the image you project...but first, go out into the hall and practice your walk. When you come back, I'll show you how wearing the right clothes will change that image."

Women make first impression judgments in seventy seconds; men make them in seven seconds.

We rushed out the door and into a dressing room, where we had secreted a change of clothes. I ripped off the false eyelashes, the miserable miniskirt, the sweater, and the hairpiece, then wiped off my makeup. I pulled a black lace dress over my head, brushed my hair into place, and quickly redid my makeup. By the time I was transformed—into a princess again—my husband was standing at the door, ready with a perfectly tailored blue business suit, his blond hair neatly combed.

We reentered the banquet room. There was a hushed silence—then applause.

It was one of my better entrances.

My headache vanished.

This personal anecdote illustrates that people do judge a book by its cover. In fact, women make first impression judgments in seventy seconds; men make them in seven seconds. We never get a second chance to make a good first impression. People guess how much money you make, how much education you have, whether they trust you, what your position in society is, how sophisticated you are—all in those first few seconds. They may not do this consciously, but subconsciously.

Ninety-five percent of our first impression is non-verbal.

That means what counts most is your handshake, body language, clothes, colors, and accessories, not personality, voice, or sincerity. Robert Pante, author of *Dressing to Win*, says, "You *always* make some kind of statement with the way you dress—powerful or inept."

In the first session of my fashion, style, and image classes, I have the students play a game. At that time no one knows anything about the other members of the class, so I have them try to identify each person's occupation from appearance alone. They seldom guess correctly. That opinion is based predominantly on what the person is wearing.

It is important for each of us to understand what image we are projecting to others. The purpose of this chapter is to identify that image. If that image is not how we think we look, or how we want to look, then it should be altered.

IMAGES

"Eat what you like, but dress for other people."
—*Benjamin Franklin*

Let us look at some obvious first impressions and how we react to them. For instance, if we see a mangy dog in the street, we will cross to the other side just to avoid it. Yet, that homeless dog may, in fact, be a warm, friendly animal looking for affection and a free meal (and a little medication).

We similarly avoid homeless people (although we empathize with their plight) as well as grungy, long-haired hitchhikers wearing torn jeans and ragged T-shirts. Though we may not want to, we judge a poorly dressed person to be beneath us, not worthy of our attention.

But clean these people up, shower them, groom them, dress them in fashionable clothes, and a revelation will take place: they will be transformed into successful and attractive-looking people.

People who *look* successful create an aura about themselves, an *image* that makes them immediately acceptable. Because of it they are able to meet others on an equal level. They are given better service in public places. They get better jobs, and they are more successful.

Just try getting a bank loan dressed in jeans and tennis shoes. The loan manager will start counting out the big bucks a lot faster if you are professionally dressed.

 Magic Trick

If you just "don't get no respect," then dress for success.

My husband has a trick that he uses whenever he needs to get down to some serious negotiating. He calls it his "power ploy." He had to use it recently when a mechanic insisted on charging him for an automobile repair that was covered by the manufacturer's warranty. Instead of arguing with the mechanic, he asked for an appointment with the service department manager.

My husband realized that the writer's "uniform" he was wearing (jeans, sweater, and tennis shoes) wasn't the right outfit for the coming confrontation. He rushed home and changed into his "power look"—dark blue sport coat, tan slacks, and striped tie. He also grabbed his mini tape recorder.

Confidently, he returned to the garage and walked into the service manager's office. He turned on the tape recorder and plopped it on the desk in front of the manager.

"I'm sure you won't mind if I record this conversation," he said.

The manager stammered, "Ah...well...I...ah...that won't be necessary."

Five minutes later, the meeting (which was quite pleasant and amicable) was over. My husband got the repairs in accordance with the warranty.

Designer Stella Mary Newton says, "We think our clothes cover us, when in fact they reveal our true personality, as we silently inspect one another." Like Morse code, clothes send out messages about our personalities.

John Malloy, in his *The Woman's Dress for Success Book*, tells us the story of a woman who was a star tax consultant when she worked in the home office, but when she went to a client's office to work on the books her sound advice was ignored. Malloy met her and immediately recognized her problem: "She was four feet, eleven inches, ninety-two pounds, blond and 'cute.' She was twenty-six and looked sixteen."

Malloy dressed her in every authority symbol her tiny frame could hold: dark suits, white blouses, silk scarves, and black-framed glasses, and had her carry a briefcase. The image change worked. Clients listened, and she was well on her way to a partnership in the firm.

My dentist, who came highly recommended, was a bit of a shock when I arrived for my first appointment. We all have mental images of medical professionals: they dress in long white coats and emanate a clinical air. The dentist I saw wore a plaid shirt, jeans, and had a scraggly mustache struggling to grow under his nose. My confidence in his ability was immediately threatened, and had he not been so highly recommended, I would have considered walking out. Yet, he performed admirably with a dentist's drill. Afterward, I asked him about his dentist's uniform.

"Oh, yeah. I tried a white coat once," he said. "I realize it's what I'm supposed to wear and that it would be better for business, but it's just not part of my personality."

Body Image

Clothing is an extension of your personality. It is also an extension of your body. If you don't like your body, you are no doubt having trouble with your clothing image.

Don't worry about your body so much. Most women are insecure about some aspect of their shape, even to the point of convincing themselves they are unattractive. Women often have imperfect self-images, images that may not be apparent to anyone but themselves. The problem is that practically every woman sets too high a standard for herself.

Okay, so we're not going to be Sophia Loren or Bo Derek, but *we are attractive*. We may not reach the level that Sharon Stone does on the beauty scale, but *we are beautiful*. We may not have started out being gorgeous, or we may have a "little" weight problem, but we must believe *we can be lovely and attractive*. So what if we are stuck with mousy hair, short legs, and big-boned bodies.

That's not our fault.

That's the figure our parents' genes gave us. All we have to do is learn how to work around our genetic hand-me-down bodies. We can change the images we project.

Don't "Weight" to be Perfect

Let's chat about fat.

Today you are told that if you are not "tall, thin, flat, and fair," with an active body shaped by exercise and cottage cheese, you are not supposed to live. The Duchess of Windsor was the one who set the tone when she said, "A woman can never be too rich or too thin." This obsession with being thin has become a symbol for happiness and well-being. And because of it, women harbor deep guilt feelings about being overweight.

"Why," you ask yourself, "why wasn't I born 100 years ago, when plumpness was stylish and men rejoiced in Rubenesque women?" Here's what an 1880 Victorian journal had to say about the ideal woman of that time:

> *Her thighs were of a largeness and fleshy plumpness seldom seen in a female. She was in fact, the very beau ideal of female beauty.*

Every era has idealized a different image of the female form. By today's standards of feminine beauty, Venus di Milo, that paragon of classic beauty since antiquity, would be judged to have figure

"A woman can never be too rich or too thin."

—The Duchess of Windsor

problems: She's a bit too hefty in the waist and hips. To give her a fashionable image with her size-16 marble shape would require a little creative styling in her clothes.

Sure, you've tried to rearrange your body fat with an exercise program, but physical workouts never were your thing. In grammar school you were the one who took "rest" while your friends took gym. You had a "cookies and milk" break instead of recess.

If dieting was as easy as

all those books say,

wouldn't one diet

be enough?

After all, waking up in the morning to a full day of liquid diet is not worth slipping into your slippers. Diet books try to make losing weight sound absurdly simple—just don't eat as much as you have been eating.

And that's the problem.

Food looks and tastes so good that over 80 percent of American women are overweight. (In California that's a thigh-to-thigh line that would reach from Los Angeles to San Francisco.) Most of these women have tried dieting, and 95 percent of them have fallen off their diets. Then gained back an extra ten pounds.

Half of the adult women in America spend one fourth of their lives dieting. They are on perpetual diets to lose five to ten pounds because they are programmed to be dissatisfied with their bodies. They eagerly try each new diet fad, and expectantly buy each new diet book. If dieting was as easy as all those books say, wouldn't one diet be enough?

A woman I know, who feels she is twenty pounds overweight, recently told me, "I dream that life will begin tomorrow, or next week, or next year, sometime after my next diet—when I have lost twenty pounds." You notice that she said after the next diet. She knows she isn't going to lose that weight.

No, I'm not recommending you go on an eating binge. A sensible intake of calories and low-fat food coupled with exercise is one of the best ways to better health. Eating healthy foods and taking vitamins can keep your skin glowing and make you radiant for the rest of your life.

Make sure you are living to be beautiful, not living to be thin.

Personal Image Enhancement

To get started on this personal image enhancement program you must first identify how you look to others. Remember, people may think of themselves as stylish, suave, and sophisticated, but because of the way they dress they may appear dowdy, careless, and lazy to others.

I had a woman come into my office at the model agency asking for a beauty consultation. She felt she was attractive enough to be a high-fashion model. Unfortunately, her image of herself was far from how others saw her. She was a tall woman, about five-ten, with beautiful auburn hair. But that's where the model qualifications ended. She was twenty pounds overweight for modeling and wore an excessively tight sheath dress that showed every bulge in her waist and hips. She had her hair done in a pony tail that came below her waist and wore false eyelashes that must have come from a costume shop.

After a long talk, this woman decided to take a basic beauty course at the agency. In one month she was able to analyze her image—and change it. She went on to take a fashion modeling course, and afterward worked as a tearoom model in hotels and restaurants. She changed her image—dramatically.

ANALYZING YOUR IMAGE

You *can* change the image you project. But first you must determine what part of your image you want to alter the most. Do you want to change

Your posture
Your personality
The way your body looks
The way your face looks
The way you dress
Your lifestyle
All of the above

Let's take a look at how others see you. Without changing the clothes you are wearing as you are reading this, stand in front of a mirror and answer these questions:

1. If you saw yourself walking down the street, what would you think?
    A. Certainly not one of my friends
    B. Wouldn't give that person a second look
    C. She's got something, but what?
    D. My, what an attractive woman
    E. I would like to meet that person

2. How would you describe the image "that person" projects?
    A. Fashionable
    B. Passably dressed
    C. Carelessly dressed
    D. Sloppy
    E. Ugh!

3. Take another hard look at yourself before you continue to walk down the street. What do you think "that person" does professionally?
    A. Librarian
    B. Store clerk
    C. Secretary
    D. Teacher
    E. Real estate agent
    F. Business executive
    G. Attorney
    H. Homemaker

4. Let's say "that person" stops to look in a store window, which gives you the opportunity to take a closer look and pick out her bad points. What would you think?

    A. Why does she wear her hair that way?

    B. A little makeup would certainly help

    C. Her posture is terrible

    D. That dress does awful things for her figure

    E. Does she have to wear those unflattering shoes?

5. While "that woman" is still looking in the window, you have time to check out her good points and how she disguises a few bad points. What do your notice?

    A. Her hair is one of her best features

    B. Her face isn't bad either

    C. She has a large waist, but it is barely noticeable in that outfit

    D. She's about twenty pounds overweight, but she disguises it well

    E. Even though she's a few pounds heavy, she looks fashionable and chic

6. The woman moves away from the window, and you take a look at the complete image she projects. What are her personality traits?

    A. Alive, vibrant

    B. Outgoing

    C. Got it all together

    D. Cautious

    E. Shy, withdrawn

7. From her appearance, what is her social status?

    A. Nob Hill matron

    B. Socialite

    C. High income

    D. Middle income

    E. Low income

    F. No income

Well, so much for what you see in "that person" on the street. Let's get down to specifics. What are *you* really like? Answer these questions honestly.

1. **My height is** (barefoot, please)
    A. Less than 5'
    B. 5' to 5'3"
    C. 5'4" to 5'6"
    D. 5'7" to 5'10"
    E. 5'11" or over

2. **My weight is** (you can fib a little here, either high or low. How much do you think you *appear to weigh* to others?)
    A. Less than 110 pounds
    B. 110 to 130
    C. 130 to 150
    D. 150 to 170
    E. Over 170

3. **My body frame is**
    A. Small
    B. Medium
    C. Large

4. **Is my weight in proportion to my body?**
    A. Yes
    B. No

5. **My figure assets** (what you need to capitalize on) **are**
    A. Bust
    B. Waist
    C. Hips
    D. Legs

6. **My figure challenges** (what you need to disguise) **are**
    A. Bust
    B. Waist
    C. Hips
    D. Legs

7. **My facial assets are**
    A. Hair
    B. Eyes
    C. Nose
    D. Mouth
    E. Complexion

8. **My facial challenges are**
    A. Hair
    B. Eyes
    C. Nose
    D. Mouth
    E. Complexion

9. **My face shape is** (Chapter Six will cover this in depth)
    A. Square
    B. Round
    C. Long
    D. Oval
    E. Heart-shaped

10. **My posture is**
    A. Good
    B. Fair
    C. Poor

11. **My body shape is**
  A. Balanced
  B. Hourglass
  C. Straight
  D. Triangular (large hips)
  E. Inverted triangle (wide shoulders or large bust)

12. **I dress to please**
  A. Myself
  B. Others
  C. Men
  D. Women

13. **I would describe my approach to dressing as**
  A. Conservative
  B. Casual
  C. Fashionable
  D. Avant-garde

14. **Other people think of me as**
  A. Motherly
  B. Chummy
  C. Respectful
  D. Standoffish
  E. Cautious
  F. Shy

15. **Other people tend to assume they know my**
  A. Background
  B. Career
  C. Education
  D. Lifestyle

16. **I believe I am "in style."**
  A. True
  B. False

17. **I am comfortable with the image I project.**
  A. True
  B. False

That's it. That's the image of the person you see in the mirror. It may not be someone you are particularly happy with, but it is someone you have to live with. You have to come to terms with the image you are now projecting, then correct the false impressions you "reflect." It's time to step out of the looking glass. It's time to create the *real you* image.

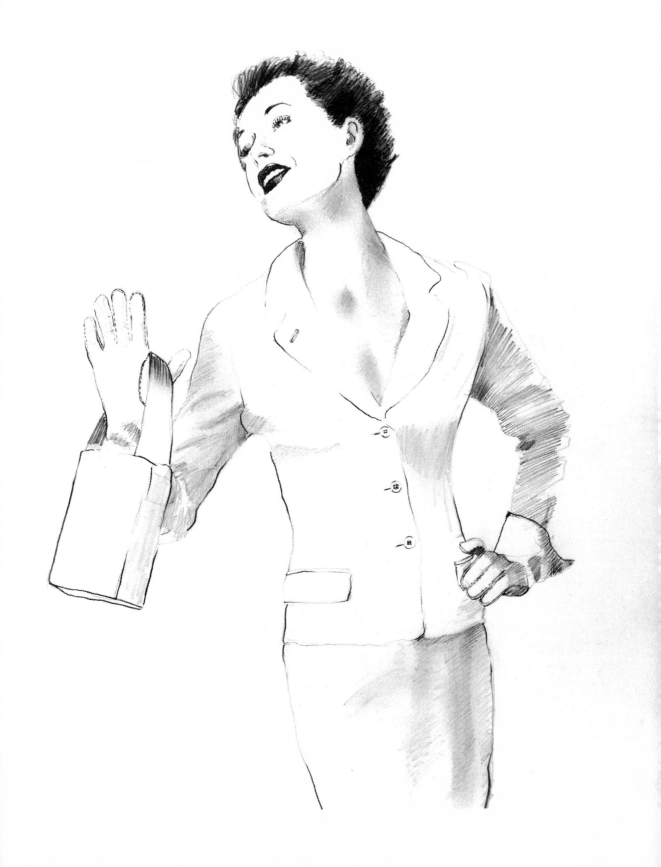

CHAPTER THREE

Body Language

From Fig Leaf to Flattery

*"Someone once told me not to lose weight or
I'd lose my personality.
Believe me, my personality
is not in my behind."*

—Oprah Winfrey

D o you ever stand with your hands clasped in front of you below your waist? In the modeling business that's called a "fig leaf." It tells the whole world that at that moment you're nervous and don't know what to do with your hands.

You don't stand around your kitchen doing the fig leaf. You do it at parties, or when you're in front of a group, or when you're having your photo taken. (Just look at some family snapshots or groups photos and see how many people are fig-leafing.)

You even see famous people doing fig leaves: presidents, actors, television personalities. One TV celebrity you've all seen is on a quiz show. She's blond and cute. She's a whiz at turning letters. She's—Vanna White! Vanna does only three things with her hands on *Wheel of Fortune*: flip cards, applaud, and do the fig leaf. When she was pregnant I was sure she'd stand with her arms at her sides. She simply clasped them under her round tummy, which looked even sillier.

What should you do with your hands? Nothing. Let them hang at your sides. It may not feel right, but it looks right. If you can't stand to have your arms dangling, then buy clothes with pockets. If you use pockets as a crutch, don't hang in them. Use a light touch. Don't jiggle change in your pockets, either.

When I was in high school I tried out for an all-school play and was cast in the part of the lead character's mother. (At that stage of my life I always seemed older—but not anymore!) At rehearsal, as I looked into the black void of the school auditorium, I was terrified. And for the first time I noticed *I had hands.* They felt like dangling lengths of rubber hose. To rid myself of these unwanted appendages, I would wring them, fold them, cross them, stuff them in my jeans, bite their fingernails, *do the fig leaf,* anything to have something to *do* with them. Finally the director, his voice booming from the darkness, yelled, "Let them hang!" I never did the fig leaf again. Neither will you.

A major step toward looking great is to evaluate your body objectively. You have to know your body and its basic silhouette. That means you're going to have to take another long look at yourself in the mirror.

Naked. (Well, perhaps with a leotard and tights.)

Look at the lines of your body. Don't worry about the challenges you're going to uncover.

The first thing to do is look at posture.

Vanna does only three things with her hands on Wheel of Fortune: *flip cards, applaud, and do the fig leaf.*

POSTURE

"Good posture identifies you as someone with something to say. People can't see your credentials—they can only see you," says Lynn Pearl, president of Executive Communications.

Poor posture is a basic figure fault in a high percentage of women. Slouching creates up to fifteen times as much pressure on your lower back as standing up straight does. When you slump your diaphragm collapses, there is less room for your lungs to expand, and the resulting shallow breathing means there is less oxygen available to nourish your body. Not only do you look anemic, but your clothes don't hang right.

I once saw two very tall women at a party; both were over six feet. One woman had obviously been unable to cope with her height. Her back was stooped and her shoulders were curved like a clam shell. She was insecure, uncomfortable, withdrawn, and her mode of dress reflected all these psychological problems. She looked dumpy.

The other woman stood up straight; she even had on three-inch high heels. She was dressed with style and exuded confidence. The men at the party looked up to her—not just literally, but as a woman who had it all together.

(Okay, ladies, while we're at it let's take a look at those men at the party. Just check out Bill, or Sam, or Joe and note the slumped shoulders, the caved-in chest, and the flabby belly hanging over the belt. Not very sexy, huh? But stand him up straight, cinch that belt properly around that stomach, not below it, and well, he'll never look like Robert Redford, but it will be an improvement.)

If you're lucky enough to have had parents who constantly reminded you to "stand up straight," then your posture is better than the average person's. I know. At five-eight I was a tall girl in my junior high school. So that I wouldn't hover over my classmates, I would slump and stick my neck out like a turtle. I began to have the silhouette of a question mark. Fortunately, my mother kept urging me (rather, yelling at me) to "straighten those shoulders!"

Remember those old cartoons of models walking around with books on their heads to improve their posture? Like those models, if you stand up straight, with your fanny tucked in, your shoulders back, and your stomach tightened, you will make an enormous difference in your appearance.

If you stand up straight, with your fanny tucked in, your shoulders back, and your stomach tightened, you will make an enormous difference in your appearance.

Magic Trick

Quick posture check: Clasp your hands behind your back, stand straight, drop your hands without moving your shoulders. That's where your shoulders should be. You can take off five to ten pounds and grow one half to one inch with good posture.

It's never too late to improve your posture. I have even taught grandmothers—and a few great-grandmothers—how to stand. It's not difficult. Here's a simple method of achieving a perfect standing position without a Marine Corps drill sergeant yelling at you to "Suck in that stomach!"

Look in that mirror. Sideways. Stand like you always do. Shoulders slumped? Stomach pooching out? Here are eight quick steps to improve what you see in the mirror:

- Chin parallel to the floor
- Shoulders back
- Diaphragm in and up
- Elbows relaxed
- Stomach muscles sucked in at all times (except when sleeping)
- Fanny tucked under; pretend you have a quarter between your buns and you don't want to drop it
- Hands relaxed at your side
- Fingertips touching your sides: no fidgets or comfort gestures, such as tugging at your ears or popping knuckles

See! You already look taller and thinner—just like magic.

Standing

Here's a special trick, a way of standing that will make you look five to ten pounds slimmer—instantly. It's called the "basic stance." Pretend there's a clock at your feet. Put your right foot at twelve o'clock, then your left foot at ten o'clock, slightly behind the right foot. Your weight should be on the left foot. Now angle your body to the left and give any observer a three-quarter view. (You can do it on opposite feet: left foot at twelve o'clock, right foot two o'clock, slightly behind the left.)

Voila! Ten pounds slimmer.

You can also modify that stance and create the same illusion. Spread the feet a little, bringing the front foot back a bit, but keep the weight on that back foot. Look at your body full-length in a mirror and see how much better it appears. Now stand with the feet spread apart in an unflattering "parade rest" position. Ugh!

Next time you see a newspaper or magazine photograph of a group of ladies posing in a line at some social function, look at the way they stand. Nine out of ten will be standing awkwardly. But one will be posed in a basic stance and will appear thinner and more attractive than the rest. Try it yourself next time you line up for a family-album portrait. When the pictures are developed, you'll be amazed how great you look.

You can use this slimming stance anywhere: at parties, in front of a group while giving a talk, shopping, at a crosswalk waiting for the stoplight to turn green—anywhere. You will look more graceful, too.

Sitting

When sitting in a chair you must also remind yourself how your body looks. Ever notice an actress on stage? She sits upright on the chair, her legs crossed at the ankle so that the line of one leg complements the other. Or, if one leg is crossed over the other knee, the upstage leg (the one further from the audience) is crossed over the other leg. That trick smooths out the lines of both legs.

You can cross your ankles by anchoring one foot on the floor and putting the other foot behind it. It's a graceful and attractive way of sitting.

You can use this slimming stance anywhere: at parties, in front of a group while giving a talk, shopping, at a crosswalk waiting for the stoplight to turn green—anywhere.

Walking

You can be perfectly coifed and dressed, but if you walk like a cow, the whole image is spoiled.

One day I was in my car waiting for a red light when a beautifully groomed professional woman, briefcase in hand, stepped from the curb into the crosswalk. That is, she was beautiful until she walked in front of my car. Actually, she didn't walk, she *clunked*, feet splayed like a duck, head forward like the prow of a ship. She was letting her body language do her talking, and it wasn't saying nice things. What a shame.

One of the most important things you "wear" is your walk.

One of the most important things you "wear" is your walk. To walk properly, men should move their feet side-by-side, like walking on narrow railroad tracks. Women should walk with their feet stepping directly in front of one another, like on a tightrope, toes pointing out no more than one inch, stride no bigger than the width of the shoulders. Arms and hands should swing at the sides, lightly touching the body, not extending like wings. This gives the illusion of slimming the lower half of the body. When walking, lead with the center of your body (two inches below the navel) and with your feet and legs, not with your head and chest. This will make you move gracefully, like royalty.

The right walk makes your hips sway from side to side so your buns will not bounce up and down like bobbing apples.

The final result of a proper walk and posture is threefold: first, you will have a slimmer look; second, your clothes will hang the way they were intended; and third, people will think that you exude confidence.

CONFIDENCE BUILDERS

Shaking Hands

When we meet someone for the first time, we shake hands. What do you think when you get a "dead mackerel" handshake? How do you feel when someone shakes the tips of your fingers? *That person has no self-esteem, no confidence.* Even if she has no self-assurance, she could fool you with a firm, friendly handshake. Like this: Grasp the other person's hand like you'd grip a tennis racquet. Put those webs (thumbs) together. This is not God creating Adam with a fingertip.

A man no longer needs to wait to see if a woman is going to shake hands; either gender may initiate a handshake. Ladies! Some men don't know this new etiquette so don't leave them wondering—stick out your hand so they'll know you intend to shake theirs. Do not offer a man four stiff, cupped fingers to deal with. Get a grip! Shake his hand.

When shaking hands, make eye contact. "Eye contact is the most remembered element in forming an impression," says Nancy Austin, co-author of *A Passion for Excellence*. Don't stare. Five to seven seconds of eye contact is enough.

Listen to the name of the person you've just met and repeat it aloud. How many times have you met someone and forgotten their name, only to have them walk up to you weeks later and remember *yours?* If you can do the same, it will show everyone what a confident person you are. (When someone's introducing you to another person, don't be shy about saying your name. It might save the person who's doing the introducing a bit of embarrassment, just in case she or he has forgotten your name.)

A man no longer needs to wait to see if a woman is going to shake hands.

Space Invasion

Have you ever talked to someone who insisted on being nose-to-nose? You back away, they step forward. You slip sideways, they circle in again. Each of us have a comfort zone of space, like a three-foot invisible bubble. We don't like to have that space invaded. Don't put your nose into someone else's space.

Compliments

If someone compliments you on your dress, do you reply, "Oh, this old thing," or "I got it on sale"? What you should say is "Thank you." Then shut up.

Ninety-five percent of communication is nonverbal. Our body language is talking loudly all the time. Even if we have butterflies, let's get them into formation and make our body "talk" the way we want it to.

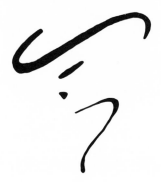

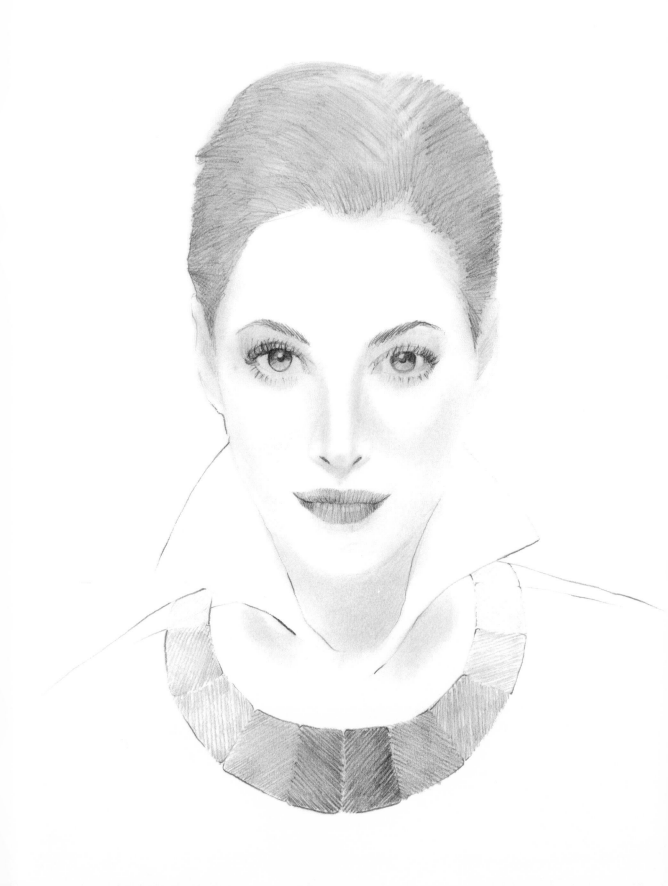

CHAPTER FOUR

Hues for You

Colors that Slim and Trim

"The only other place I can work is to enlist in the army, as khaki is a smashing color with my reddish hair and beige skin."

—Erma Bombeck

Color is everywhere. Color is the first thing we have to deal with when we get up in the morning, and the last thing we look at when we turn out the lights. (That is, unless you are one of the 20 percent who dream in color.)

The colors we wear communicate a lot about ourselves to others. We identify the "blond" who works at the bank, the executive who wears the "blue" blazer. (We also make immediate, automatic decisions about whether we like or dislike a person simply from the color he or she wears.)

Why are we programmed to like or dislike certain colors? Do we get all the little cells together in the brain and vote on it? Does one cell say, "Hey, this color really excites me!" only to have the next cell reply, "Naw, that color's boring"?

Actually, we don't have any vote in the matter. You see, when a color fills your field of vision, the pituitary

gland, which works like a third eye, takes over. It is totally depen-
dent on your brain and doesn't know anything about your likes and
dislikes. Instead, it automatically sends out a chemical signal to the
adrenal gland in the kidneys, which in turn secrets epinephrine or
adrenaline, which causes certain responses in the body. A response
to color is automatic and can even cause you to breathe faster, your
blood pressure to increase, and your heart to beat rapidly. All because you saw a color.

Different colors send different messages, causing people to
respond to each color differently. The "color language" works in
strange ways.

COLOR TRICKS

Let's take a look at the different colors and discover how
they affect our reactions.

Pale blue is one of the greatest diet-enhancement colors. If
you want to lose weight, I recommend you hang a blue bulb over
your dining room table (the kind used to illuminate a garden palm
tree). Just let it glow over your plate. You're not going to eat blue la-
sagna or blue vanilla ice cream. There is a weight-reducing spa not
far from me that uses blue place mats, blue napkins, and blue rims
on their dishes to dull the appetite. It works.

Navy blue is the power color and signifies stability and respect. If you ever go to court, make sure your lawyer is wearing a
blue suit. It was in A.D. 431 that the Virgin Mary was first illustrated
wearing a blue cloak, and she has worn one ever since. In the garment industry, 80 percent of all fibers are dyed in blue tones.

Blue is also a calming color. (If your dentist doesn't wear a
blue smock, ask him to.) We are tranquilized when we look at blue.

Red is exciting and stimulating. It's one of the favorite colors of women all over the world. Nancy Reagan chose it as her favorite color. She even appeared on the cover of *Time* outfitted in red. It is not the greatest color for diets—or for the pocketbook. In the presence of red, you eat longer and pay more for your food. Some of the most exclusive restaurants have red decor.

Men have a natural preference for yellow-based (warm) reds, like a tomato. Infant boys will stare much longer at a yellow-based red than a blue-based (cool) red. A female baby's attention is held by blue-based reds, like a watermelon.

If you are trying to get a man's attention, just hope you are in the right color season (spring or autumn) to wear a yellow-based red outfit. If your boyfriend starts breathing heavily, it may not be your clever repartee that is turning him on, but your dress.

Pink is the "tasty" color. We think candy and pastries taste better if they come in pink tissue. If you made a dessert that didn't come out just right, put it on a pink plate. You'll get raves. (A candy company tested this color theory. They got a group of people together and put half of them in pink booths, the other half in green booths. Then they served them the same candy. The people in the pink booths thought the candy was wonderful; those in the green booths thought the candy was nauseating.)

Medium bright pink is also recommended as a calming color. Prisoners put in a pink room have had their aggressive behavior subdued—for brief periods of time. But if you have a hyperactive daughter, I wouldn't suggest painting her bedroom a Pepto-Bismol pink. You can't be surrounded by this color for a long period of time; fifty minutes is enough. After that it loses its effectiveness as a tranquilizing agent. Perhaps you could paint the bathroom pink; then if you are feeling a little edgy, just hole up for a few minutes.

Yellow is cheerful and warm, but because it is the most intense color for the eye to process, yellow can create anxiety. It can be an indicator of something dangerous, like a bumblebee or a warning sign on the highway. Yellow should be used in small amounts or places where you don't spend a lot of time, such as patios. Obviously, the color is not good for kitchens. Use yellow as an accent color in your wardrobe.

Gold means glamour and wealth.

Purple is royal. The American Revolution decreed that the wearing of purple was undemocratic (and even hinted that it was not masculine). A purple jogging suit is okay in California, but don't ask your husband to wear one if he's from Kansas. Women wear purple. Be careful. If you're pear-shaped, you may look like an eggplant.

In the presence of green,

people feel secure

and cared for.

Green is coolness. In the presence of green, people feel secure and cared for. (Money is green.) Green is not a good color to wear in business, unless you are a recreational camp counselor. When green turns to forest green, it appeals to upper socioeconomic levels only.

Brown is also a color that makes people feel secure.

White means purity, and indicates refinement and delicacy. Only in recent times has it indicated virginity. Nothing looks more elegant at a formal ball than a white gown.

Orchid is a nausea-inducing color. Don't go throwing your orchid blouses away; you're not going to make your husband sick. But don't paint your living room this color. Have you ever seen a room on a ship or an airliner painted in orchid colors?

Orange is orange, like pumpkins, or oranges from a tree. Orange is a second-class color. It isn't intimidating to anyone. Would you ever think of wearing an orange dress to a formal occasion? If you go to a very exclusive Ritz-Carlton hotel, the interior may be decorated in forest green. If you add orange to it you have a Holiday Inn. Just take a look at the next Howard Johnson's restaurant you enter.

Gray is another relaxing color. One can create longer and be more productive in a gray room.

Turquoise is an excellent attention-getter. If you want people to look at you, wear turquoise.

The point of understanding the psychology of color is to use it to help create the image you want for a particular situation—job hunting, parties, meetings. Are you trying to look powerful, or feminine? Color is one of the most important illusions in the magic of looking great.

Slenderizing with Color

Remember the day you went out and felt wonderful? You thought you looked great. Then a friend came up and said, "Gee, do you feel all right?" Why did she say that? Why did you look so sick? You probably had on the wrong color, one that made you look like you'd just been exhumed.

Then there was the day you dressed up in that new pink outfit and went to the luncheon, and one of the ladies remarked, "Oh, my dear, you better go light on the strawberry shortcake." Why? Well, that pink dress made you look like a party balloon.

Black carries the most visual weight of any color.

My husband has an instant slenderizing trick. If he's put on an extra inch around the waist, he goes for his black shirt or dark blue sweater. He has a round face, and everyone remembers him a bit heavier than he is. With a black shirt on, he invariably hears, "Hey, you've lost a little weight, haven't you?"

Let's take a look at the basic color **black**, which carries the most visual weight (no pun intended) of any color. We wear it as a signal of refinement, of sophistication, of power. (It wasn't that many centuries ago that black meant terror, as in the black plague or a pirate ship's flag.) We also wear it to create a visual image of slenderness.

Black or dark colors make your form appear to retreat and look slimmer.

White or lighter colors act in reverse. They appear to advance and make you look larger.

The idea is to mix the light and dark colors to balance your body proportions. At a recent event I couldn't help noticing a wide-shouldered, large-bosomed woman who was wearing a brilliant white blouse that hung to her waist, and black pants that narrowed dramatically at her ankles. She looked like a dagger stuck in the floor. The light-hued blouse emphasized her upper body portions, and the black pants made her already slender hips almost invisible. She needed to reverse the colors to balance her act.

 Magic Trick

Large prints increase body size, but a solid bright color that runs in one continual line from neck to hemline is slimming because it diverts attention from your body to your total balanced look.

THE SEASONAL COLOR SYSTEM

Wearing your own seasonal colors will coordinate your overall look. Seasonal colors will also flatter your skin and draw attention to your face and away from your body. The right colors will make your face glow with vitality.

Not long ago I went with a friend to an afternoon party. She was decked out in a black-and-white print dress that was all wrong for her. She is a Summer person and should never wear black next to her face. Her face looked drawn, tired, and wrinkled, and she appeared to be every bit of her forty-two years. I saw her again the next day. She had on a baby-blue outfit and looked refreshed, healthy, and at least five years younger.

Magic Trick

For an instant facelift, wear colors that are in your season. Wrinkles and blemishes will blend into your skin and be less visible. Teeth will get whiter and eyes brighter.

To achieve that instant facelift, you must know your color season. Learning is quite painless. First let's take a look at the two basic color groups: cool and warm.

Cool and Warm

The basis of the color system is cool and warm color tones. First, decide whether you have a warm skin color, or a cool skin color.

Cool skin tones are white, rosy pink, olive, or charcoal brown.
Warm skin tones are peachy pink, golden tan, or golden brown.

To do a simple color analysis and determine whether you have a cool or warm skin tone, you must first remove all your makeup. If you have changed your hair color or tinted it, cover your hair with a scarf. What is left to look at is your true skin color. If you have a sun tan (let's hope not), you still have the same skin tone, it's just a little darker. (If you are sunburned—heaven forbid!—wait until the red is gone.) As you get older your skin tone may fade a little, but it won't change seasons.

You will need two pieces of material about the size of a small towel. One must be in a warm orange tone, like the color of a pumpkin, the other a cool pink tone, like bright fuchsia. If you don't have these two colors in your wardrobe, get material swatches from a fabric shop.

Take one of the color swatches and hold it under your chin

and look in a mirror. (Make sure that you are in natural light.) Then take the other swatch and do the same.

Does the warm orange color turn your skin yellow or sallow? Or does it smooth and blend facial lines and make your skin glow? If it looks vibrant, then you have warm skin tones.

Do the same with the cool pink swatch. If your skin appears complemented by this color, you have cool skin tones. There are more people in the cool category than warm.

If you have difficulty judging your skin tone (one out of 200 women is color blind, one out of twelve men is), then ask a friend to take a look at your face with the two different color tones.

Remember: *the basis of the seasonal color system is these warm and cool tones.*

There are two warm seasons—**Spring** and **Autumn**.

There are two cool seasons—**Summer** and **Winter**.

What season are you?

What are your colors?

HAVING YOUR COLORS ANALYZED

Having your colors done professionally can be a valuable aid in choosing your wardrobe. Color analysts drape you in color swatches, peer at every pore in your face, then determine exactly what season you are—Spring, Autumn, Summer, or Winter—and what colors go perfectly with your natural skin tone.

This should help keep you from being a fashion victim. You'll know what colors flatter you, and you won't have to try on clothes with colors that don't. You'll have your own personal palette of colors.

Humorist Erma Bombeck once decided she was the last woman in North America to be "draped," and so she succumbed to "having her colors done." After she completed her color analysis, Bombeck was classified as an Autumn. She wrote: "I realize there are only two things in my closet I can wear with confidence; a beige T-shirt and a nightgown that came out gray when I washed it with a pair of boy's trousers. The rest can go."

Unlike Erma Bombeck, who said she "glowed in khaki," I look like a reject from a terrorist group in that color. I am a Winter person—but I love khaki. And—I wear it! I realize that my personal color palette is not an absolute. Khaki may be bad for me, but I can wear it if I keep the color away from my face. I wear scarves and accessories that *are* in my color palette.

It was the fashion industry that first made me fall in love with khaki when years ago the designers decreed that khaki was the new color for *everyone*. Unfortunately, it only flatters 8 percent of the population.

A good example of what *not* to do with color are the jackets that Century 21 realtors have to wear. First of all, autumn gold is a bad business color; and second, it only looks good on eight out of 100 agents. That means the other ninety-two appear too sick to sell you a house.

Network sportscasters wear blue sport coats, either in a cool blue or a warm blue to match their skin tones. They look great on camera.

The seasonal color system is not a new idea. I know. It was taught to me in the late 1950s when I was enrolled in "charm school" in Spokane, Washington. Actually, the color system began in the 1930s when an artist, Johannes Itten, who was a leading colorist of the Bauhaus school, developed what is known as the Seasonal Color Theory. Itten observed that each season of the year has its own definite color scheme, and individual artists used those palettes. Color coordinators in the fashion and cosmetic industry eventually applied this concept to skin color.

We are surrounded by color, and must make hundreds of color decisions each day; 60 percent of a first impression has to do with what color a person is wearing. (After all, only your head and arms stick out of these colors.) Obviously, color selection is the single most important thing we can do each day for our grooming. Yet we all make terrible mistakes. How many mistakes? Answer these questions *yes* or *no* and let's see:

The seasonal color system began in the 1930s when artist Johannes Itten observed that each season has its own color scheme.

	Yes	No
Do you constantly buy clothes but have nothing to wear?	☐	☐
Is shopping for clothes a chore?	☐	☐
Have you purchased any clothes lately that you realized were a mistake?	☐	☐
Do you pack two suitcases for a trip and wish you could get along with one?	☐	☐
Do you have trouble figuring out what accessories to wear (purses, brief-cases, and watches included)?	☐	☐
Do you have doubts when buying makeup colors?	☐	☐
Are you uncomfortable in surroundings such as your house or car?	☐	☐

If you answered "yes" to most of these questions, you don't understand seasonal colors. It's time to learn.

COLOR COORDINATION

You are born color-coordinated with a specific skin tone that will stay with you as long as you live. Nature was very good to us, but then we proceed to mess it up. We wear the wrong hair color, the wrong lipstick and nail polish, and worst of all, the wrong color clothes. Here's a little story to show you how it works.

A Fairy Tale

Once upon a time, there was a sweet little girl and her name was Eloise. She had light brown hair, pink-toned skin, and blue eyes, all color-coordinated by nature. She was a perfect Summer.

Eloise was a happy, playful little girl until she turned fourteen. Then, to be like her friends, she decided to dye her hair half orange, half hot pink. The hot pink side wasn't too bad, but the orange side…ugh!

Eloise grew out of that, thank goodness, but when she reached twenty she decided her hair was mousy. She bleached it brassy blond. She also went to a clothes sale and bought a great dress that had been $100 and was marked down to $5. Never mind that it was orange and made her look like a Halloween pumpkin.

She took the pumpkin dress home and, to her dismay, discovered it made her skin look like she had jaundice. She hurried back to the department store, marched up to the makeup counter, and cried to the clerk: "Help!" The clerk couldn't have been happier, because Eloise, in order to complement the orange dress, needed everything from foundation to eye shadow to lipstick. Eloise spent the $95 she'd saved on her sale dress on makeup. She still looked like a pumpkin.

Then Eloise had her thirty-fifth birthday. In the mirror she saw a gray hair. Horrors! She immediately dyed her hair jet black (which would have been fine if she had been a Winter person). Soon Eloise turned forty-five, and the jet black hair made her wrinkles look like rivers. She felt miserable. She looked in the mirror and cried, "Help!"

And the mirror whispered softly, "Color.…"

So Eloise decided to have her colors analyzed.

The color consultant explained she was a Summer person, and suggested she have her hair highlighted cool blond. The color consultant showed Eloise the colors that flattered her pink-toned skin and had her throw away the orange dress—immediately. (It had been cluttering up her closet for over twenty years.) The consultant also advised her to toss away the warm beige makeup foundation, copper eye shadow, and orange lipstick.

Eloise did what she was told and looked younger and felt better than she had for years. And she lived happily ever after.

The end.

Are you like Eloise? If so, you need to know your colors. The following is only a guide, not a rule. There are dozens of shades in each of your colors, so use it as an aid; do not try to match colors specifically. For more information on color, I suggest you read Carol Jackson's book, *Color Me Beautiful*, or go to a certified color analyst.

Warm

Spring A Spring's seasonal colors are warm, crisp, clear, and fresh. Think of trees budding a bright, clear green, and flowers blooming, like yellow daffodils and red tulips. All Spring colors will have yellow undertones.

Your **skin tone** is:
Peach · Golden · Ivory

Your **eye color** is:
Clear blue · Aqua · Clear green · Golden brown

Your **hair color** is:
Golden blond · Auburn · Golden brown
Golden gray · Red · Strawberry blond

A Spring person should have golden blond hair, never beige blond. Springs do best by remaining some shade of blond all their lives, as they usually don't gray well. But they can look years younger longer.

Your best colors are orange-red and bright yellow to soft delicate peach. Oranges range from light fruit tones to rust. Violet shades are light to medium, and white is creamy. Camels and tans are of a medium shade. Browns are golden, blues are clear, gray is also clear, but warm. Avoid dark colors, such as black and blue-red.

Basic colors are vanilla, light tan, camel, brown, rust, dune gray, and colonial blue.

Several famous Spring personalities are Julie Andrews, Goldie Hawn, Sissy Spacek, Debbie Reynolds, and Daryl Hannah.

Autumn Think earthy, of tree leaves turning their golden colors—rust, copper, or olive. These colors are warm, like Spring, but more muted, dustier. All have yellow undertones.

> Your **skin tone** is:
> Ivory · Peach · Golden · Beige

> Your **eye color** is:
> Brown · Amber · Hazel · Blue-green

> Your **hair color** is:
> Red · Golden blond or brown · Copper
> Black (charcoal) · Golden gray

Autumns usually need some tinting during graying, but it can be an attractive gray.

Autumns look best in browns, beiges, and tans that have a golden tone. Gray must be a brown-gray. Blues are rich teal, turquoise, and rich violets. Greens are bright to olive, with golden tones. Golds, oranges, and rust colors are the right ones. Avoid black, blue-reds, and pink.

Basic colors are creamy white, light beige, gold, browns, rust, olive.

Some famous Autumn people are Shirley MacLaine, Ann-Margret, Stephanie Powers, Carol Burnett, Sigourney Weaver.

Remember: Autumn and Spring are related, as they are warm-toned.

Cool

Winter Think of snow. Think of frosty, dramatic colors that are clear and pure, like black and white. Winter colors are strong, definite, and have blue undertones. Pastels are icy.

Your **skin tone** is:
White · Rosy · Olive · Charcoal brown · Sallow

Your **eye color** is:
Dark blue · Gray-blue · Dark brown · Green

Your **hair color** is:
Black · Salt and pepper · Silver gray
White · Dark brown

Winters gray beautifully, naturally.

The best colors for a Winter person are pure white, black, and navy. Blues are clear or icy. Turquoise and purple are vivid jewel tones. Yellow is clear and lemon. Burgundy is a deep color. Red is blue-red, beiges are rosy or taupe. Avoid orange colors.

Basic colors are icy, white, light gray, charcoal gray, black, navy, taupe, burgundy, forest green.

Here are a few famous Winter people: Elizabeth Taylor, Cher, Sally Field, Lynda Carter, Joan Collins, Demi Moore.

Summer Think of a rose in full bloom, a softer color than a spring bud. More muted and dusty than winter's stark, bright colors.

Your **skin tone** is:
Pink · Rosy · Pale beige

Your **eye color** is:
Bright blue · Soft brown · Gray-blue · Gray-green
Gray · Hazel

Your **hair color** is
Beige blond · Brown · Mousy

A Summer person who has blond hair will be beige, never golden. Because Summer people often have mousy brown hair, they are ideal candidates for highlighting.

A Summer's best colors are soft and grayed whites, rose-browns, and rose-beiges. Grays are blue-toned and soft. Aqua is medium to light. Purples are like soft plums or lavenders. Pinks are blue-toned. Yellow is soft and light. Avoid oranges, golds, or black.

Basic colors are off-white, taupe, navy, burgundy, powder blue, blue-gray, rose-beige.

Here are some famous Summer people: Queen Elizabeth, Candice Bergen, Caroline Kennedy, Princess Diana, Barbra Streisand, Jessica Lange, Glenn Close.

Once you have discovered your color palette, remember that you may look even better in some colors within that palette than others. That is because there are light and dark shades, pastels and bright colors in all seasons.

Now that you have discovered what season you are, you will likely see garments in your wardrobe that are the wrong color. They are probably the things you wear least, so you might want to do some tossing. If not, you can still wear them. Just keep the color away from your face. If it is a skirt or pants that are in the wrong color, match them with a blouse or sweater that is flattering. If it is a dress, fill in the neck area with a scarf or jewelry in the proper color. In your future apparel purchases, you'll be happier if you stick closer to your color palette.

Magic Trick

If you add a second or third color when dressing, repeat the color at least once. The easiest way would be with belt, shoes, or earrings.

Jewelry

Winter and **Summer** people look better in silver, platinum, or rose gold, rather than yellow gold. This doesn't mean you have to throw away your wedding ring or all your gold jewelry because it is the wrong color. Try mixing the metals. Get a gold and silver watch. Wear a combination of gold and silver chains. If you are making a statement with large costume jewelry, use silver. If you're buying lamé, make it silver; it reflects well on your skin. Your pearls should be white or rosy, never yellow toned.

Spring and **Autumn** people look best in golds, coppers, and bronzes. Pearls should have a golden cast.

 Magic Trick

By using the right colors you will need fewer accessories because they will blend with your wardrobe. *Use the color system to simplify your life.*

Try using one of your basic colors in choosing a billfold, checkbook cover, briefcase, and even a key ring. Camels and browns for Spring and Autumn; taupe, raisin brown, burgundy, and black for Summer and Winter. When you're buying a gift for someone, male or female, consider what season they might be. That way you'll choose a color they like, not necessarily one you like.

Many people naturally decorate their homes in colors in which they look good and feel comfortable.

If you have children, listen to their color preferences. They may be different seasons than you are. In my own family I have an Autumn husband, a Summer daughter, and a Winter son.

Even when you buy a car, consider your season. Why not choose one you'll look good in instead of a car that makes you look sick? Have fun with color and make it work for you.

THE COLOR MARKETING GROUP

Unfortunately, the colors that we know we look the best in are not always the fashion craze. What's "in" for this fall or next spring may be totally out of your color spectrum. Why? Where do designers get the colors they use each season? Do they huddle together in a pink-hued room and decide that brilliant pink will look smashing on *everyone* next season? No, it's more programmed than that.

Colors are created commodities. Each year the Color Marketing Group, a Virginia-based color cartel, comprised of 1,500 members, makes a decision on what colors all of us will be wearing, driving around in, sitting on, or looking at. (Remember those avocado refrigerators of the Sixties, and the mauve motel rooms of the Seventies? That's the Color Marketing Group at work.) An elite group of qualified decorators and fashion designers, they combine their ideas and choose colors for the future. The new colors are selected three years in advance, as dyes and pigments must be made and distributed to manufacturers. The reason the Color Marketing Group goes to all this trouble? Primarily, to create order in the manufacturing world from the 6 million color choices available. But also, to stimulate sales, kind of a programmed "color obsolescence."

Where do designers get the colors they use each season?

The company that made your hot-pink shoes didn't call up the two designers who made your pink belt and matching pink handbag and say, "Hey, what are you making tomorrow?" They buy the colors each year in a packet, and each little packet costs about $1,500. That sounds like a terrible price, but not for the Ford Motor Company, which must pick the latest colors for exterior paint and interior upholstery, or Cannon Mills, which makes a whole batch of new towels based on what the Color Marketing Group has decreed.

Your problem, as a consumer, is to decide whether the new colors are right for you. You must know whether a color is in your season. You must know whether you have cool or warm skin tones. You must know whether you are a Spring or Autumn, a Winter or Summer person.

The point of knowing your seasonal colors is that it not only makes your skin, teeth, and eyes look great, but it simplifies your wardrobe. You will need fewer shoes and handbags because everything will blend. Obviously, it is more economical using seasonal colors.

Colors add that extra magic touch to your look, instantly.

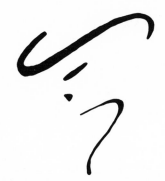

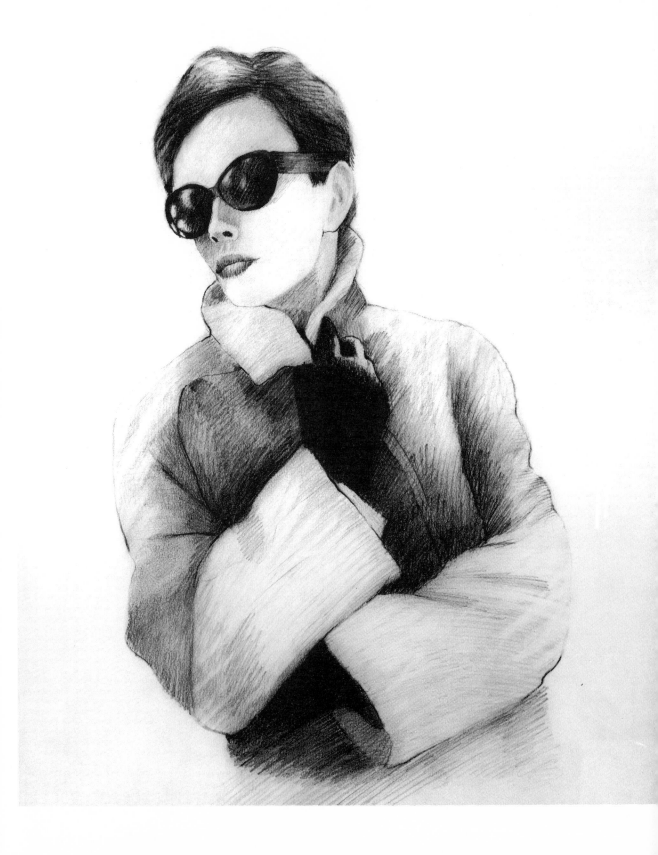

CHAPTER FIVE

Facing the Facts

New Wrinkles in Skin Care

Slip on a shirt
Slap on a hat
Slop on suntan lotion

—*Australian Beach Sign*

Lynn J. Parentini, a writer for *Energy Times* magazine, likened our skin to a "head-to-toe suit of armor," one that protects us against nature's "harsh environment." But like a suit of armor that can rust if not properly oiled, shined, and protected, our skin must be guarded against the abuses we thrust upon it: smoking, lack of exercise, too much alcohol, and worst of all, the sun. Unlike that armor, which can be discarded when it is rent with dents and covered with rust, our skin has to last a lifetime. Parentini went on to wonder how our skin would look if treated roughly:

> Leathered and worn or smooth or fresh? Unfortunately our skin doesn't come with care instructions. Like a fine silk blouse that says "do not bleach, and do not dry with excessive heat" the care label of your skin would read "do not go into the sun unprotected." If you follow these instructions carefully, the fibers of your skin would not become prematurely worn.

67

Now there is nothing wrong with aging. We have to remember that it is not a disease, but a natural process. It's like a fine bottle of wine; we as individuals should improve with age. Yet even with wine you must follow special care instructions so that the vintage wine doesn't turn to vinegar.

To have nice skin, *pick your parents carefully*, use sun screen, and follow a good skin care regimen. Here's how to make your skin last that lifetime.

SKIN CARE

Let's think of your face as an artist's canvas. Obviously, an artist can't paint on a dirty canvas, and neither can you apply makeup to skin that isn't properly cleansed and moisturized. Each of us has a different canvas to work with. Here are the four different skin types:

- Dry
- Oily
- Combination (oily in the T-zone of your nose and forehead, dry on the cheeks)
- Normal

No matter what type of skin you have, there are four steps to good skin care:

1. Cleanse
2. Stimulate
3. Protect
4. Moisturize

1. Cleanse

Cleaning your face thoroughly is one of the most important ways to maintain a good complexion. All beauty experts agree—don't go to bed with your makeup on! You must get all the dirt, grime, and old makeup off your face every single day.

How do you clean your face? With the same soap you use on the rest of your body? I hope not, as common bath soaps will dry your skin. If you do use soap, use one with a glycerin base or one made especially for the face. These soaps cost more, so save them for your face only.

You can use cleansing lotion, either liquid or cream, followed by a freshner or toner. Never use astringents on your face unless your skin is oily. They contain alcohol and dry the skin.

Magic Trick

Try using these two inexpensive drugstore products: Cetaphil, which is recommended by many plastic surgeons for cleansing the face no matter what type skin; and Brite-Life Glycerin and Artificial Rosewater as a toner. My personal favorites for years!

---

2. Stimulate

The only products on the market today that truly help wrinkles are Retin A, alpha hydroxy acids, and sunscreen.

Retin-A (derived from vitamin A) won't improve expression lines from furrows or sagging skin, but it can improve crow's feet, fine wrinkling around the eyes, fine crinkled lines on the backs of the hands, age or liver spots, and vertical lines around the lips. It will also lighten freckles and age spots and minimize large pores.

Retin-A is a prescription drug and requires the approval of a dermatologist. It is expensive (unless you go to Mexico, where no prescription is necessary). It is also strong and can dry the skin. Discuss all the pros and cons of its use with your dermatologist.

A newer and more exciting product is now on the market: alpha-hydroxy acid (AHA), a less potent way to mimic the benefits of Retin-A. No prescription is required, and it is less expensive. AHAs are naturally occurring non-toxic substances derived from sugar. Common sources are sugar cane (glycolic acid) and sour milk (lactic acid). These natural products contain substances known as alpha-hydroxy acids, which are ideal for cosmetic use.

AHAs exfoliate by weakening the "glue" that holds dead cells together in the skin's outermost layers. While doctors use them in high concentrations (30–70 percent) to perform deep-skin peels that remove scars and superficial wrinkles, cosmetic companies use AHAs at low strength (1–15 percent). AHAs are generally believed to be effective only if the concentration is above 5 percent. An inexpensive drugstore brand, Alpha Hydrox, labels its cream at 8 and 10 percent. Many companies have AHA products but don't list the concentration.

AHAs benefit oily skin by helping remove dead cells that clog pores and cause skin breakouts. They benefit dry skin by sloughing off cells that impede moisturization.

Apply the product to clean, damp skin. Damp skin absorbs more acid because water creates spaces between skin cells through which the acid moves easily. Conversely, if you find the product stings, wait until your face is dry before applying. You can apply makeup over it after it's dry, but I suggest you use it only at night.

AHAs exfoliate by weakening the "glue" that holds dead cells together in the skin's outermost layers.

3. Protect

No sun tan is healthy. Sun may be good for tomatoes, but it is not good for your skin. A tan is a traumatic experience for the skin to undergo. Eighty percent of aging is caused by the sun. The sun is also responsible for skin cancers. When you tan or sunburn you break down the elastic fibers and collagen that give skin its tone and resilience. Then come the wrinkles and sagging skin.

I remember when I was in college everyone wanted that "healthy" look from a golden bronze tan. I would spend hours on the roof of the sorority studying in my swimsuit, gaining that glorious tan. My parents had a home on the lake, and in the summer I would water ski and tan on the front lawn. And a suntan lotion? Never! I wanted to tan—fast. Some of my friends even used baby oil, mixed with a little iodine for a quick tan. It was like being basted in the sun. Fortunately, those tanning days were short lived, as I never really did like to spend all that time in the sun. It was too hot.

Tanning is the body's way of attempting to shield itself from ultraviolet rays by increasing melanin. Dark skin naturally has more melanin than light skin. Skin that is repeatedly browned looks up to twenty years older than protected body parts.

Instead of thinking of a tan as healthy, think of it as visible evidence of injury. Sun damage is cumulative. Sun ages skin by drying outer layers, thickening the skin, and breaking down fibers. Sun encourages cancer and cataracts. How many times have you seen women with crepe-paper necks and mottled skin on the chest, with deep wrinkles from years of constant sun exposure?

Tanning salons have four times as much ultraviolet radiation as the sun.

Tanning salons have four times as much ultraviolet radiation as the sun. You can end up looking like a leather purse.

UVB rays are the ones that burn. They are the deadliest from 10:00 A.M. to 3:00 P.M. You need a sun block lotion with a SPF (sun protection factor) of at least 15. (Inexpensive sunscreen is just as effective as expensive.) If you normally burn in ten minutes, the tanning lotion will "buy" ten times the time, or 150 minutes.

UVA rays are the aging rays. Longer in length than UVB, there is no SPF number by which to measure them. They sneak up on you, under an umbrella (sand reflects 20 percent of UV rays), in the water (75 percent of UV penetrates up to thirty feet of water), on the ski slopes (snow reflects 85 percent of UV), and even through your clothes (a cotton T-shirt lets in 6 percent of UV rays).

Dark-skinned people are not immune to sun damage. Dark skin gives a person an advantage of perhaps an hour over someone with lighter skin.

NASA researchers have discovered that the ozone layer is thinning twice as fast as they previously thought, so you need year-round protection. In the fall, UVB (burning rays) are fewer than in the summer; but there is no seasonal change in UVA (aging rays) that damage the skin's collagen support structure.

Cloudy days? About 80 percent of UV rays penetrate clouds. Ten minutes a day of this kind of exposure for a year adds up to more UV radiation than a week on the beach.

Researchers say 80 percent of our yearly UV exposure is due to seemingly harmless activity such as walking from house to car, even on dull, cloudy days.

To those who say sun is beneficial because of the doses of vitamin D it provides, I answer, yes, but you get enough vitamin D from simply walking around daily.

Sixty years ago the lifetime risk of developing malignant melanoma was one in 1,500. Today it is 1 in 105 and the incidence of this (sometimes fatal) cancer is growing rapidly in women under forty. Women spend thousands on facelifts and collagen injections when simple sun protection would stave off skin damage. Although sun damage is cumulative, it is never too late to start using protection. You can partially reverse the damage no matter how old you are.

Sunscreen must be considered *basic* skin care. Like the armor of a medieval knight going into battle, sunscreen is your protective armor. Dermatologists say, "Always wear an SPF-15 or higher." (Remember, SPF measures only UVB blockage. To block UVA, look for a product labeled "broad spectrum" that contains ingredients such as benzophenone, avobenzone, or oxybenzone.)

Sunscreens begin their work through a chemical reaction with the skin cells. Since it takes a while, apply the sunscreen an hour before going into the sun. Wear your SPF-15 wherever your skin shows (lower arms, hands, neck, face). During water sports, use a sunscreen that is waterproof, and reapply as necessary. Teach your children to put on sunscreen every morning when they brush their teeth. Babies under six months should not use sunscreen. Usually half of the damage our skin receives in our lifetime is done by the time we reach eighteen, because children are outdoors more than adults.

Suntan in a Bottle So, despite what you know, you just must have a tan. Perhaps you're going on a Caribbean cruise and want to lounge around the deck pool under an umbrella looking like one of the bikini-clad extras from "Baywatch." That's fine. Just

Sixty years ago

the lifetime risk of

developing malignant

melanoma was

1 in 1,500.

Today it is

1 in 105.

buy your suntan in a bottle. No, it won't turn you orange (like old-fashioned early products).

The active ingredient found in self-tanners is a protein called dihydroxacetone (DHA), which has been safely used by Coppertone since 1966. A self-tanner's color intensity is determined by the amount of DHA it contains.

DHA works by interacting with the amino acids in the skin's dead surface cells, creating a tanlike color in three hours. As the dead cells are sloughed off over the next three to six days, the color fades naturally. "DHA has no effect on living cells," says Frank Akin, Ph.D., senior director of research at Schering-Plough Health Care Products, which makes Coppertone. "It's strictly a cosmetic product."

Skin that gets its color from self-tanners is not protected by increased melanin levels. It still needs SPF-15 sunscreen. Buy a self-tanner with SPF-15.

To apply, start with clean, well-exfoliated skin. Rough spots, knees, and elbows can darken unevenly. Allow time for the product to dry before putting on clothes; it could stain. Wash hands with soap and water immediately after application. Orange palms are a bottle tan giveaway.

Reapply every three to six days to maintain your tan. To deepen color apply every three or four hours until you achieve the desired color.

Alcohol is a diuretic, which draws water out of the tissue, leaving the skin dull and dry.

"Puff, Puff, Puff That Cigarette." Another thing that prematurely ages the skin is smoking. It causes blood vessels in your eyes to constrict, affects the color of your skin, and forms tiny aging lines.

"Make Mine a Double." Alcohol in excess over-dilates blood vessels and can weaken capillary walls to the point of rupture, causing splotches under the skin. Alcohol is a diuretic, which draws water out of the tissue, leaving the skin dull and dry. Help your skin from the inside with vitamins, good diet, and by drinking lots of water. Water flushes toxins out through the pores.

Exercise boosts blood circulation and increases blood volume so the skin gets more nutrients and oxygen. Perspiration flushes out dirt and impurities. It raises skin temperature, which speeds up the production of collagen, keeping the skin younger looking.

4. Moisturize

Water or moisture in your skin is what keeps it beautiful and youthful. As skin ages it loses moisture, so use a moisturizing face cream at night unless you are using an AHA product. Also moisturize in the morning after applying sunscreen, or do one step and buy a moisturizer with at least 15 SPF as an ingredient. A reasonably priced drugstore product is Neutrogena Moisture SPF 15 untinted. Your makeup foundation will go on smoothly and evenly over it. The cream also keeps makeup and air pollutants out of your pores.

As your years increase until you are a "classic," you will be ecstatic that you protected your skin, especially when you go to that thirty-year class reunion and you're the youngest-looking grad there.

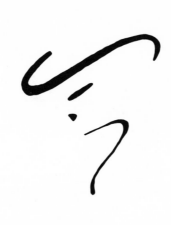

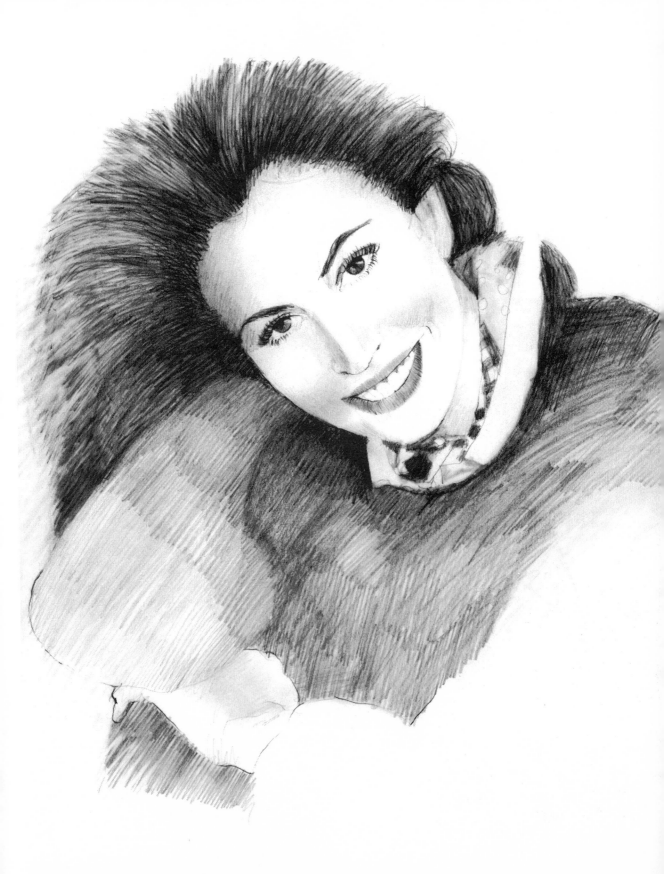

CHAPTER SIX

Makeup Magic

The Trick of Putting on Your Best Face

"I think I look like a pig without my makeup."

—Boy George

All of us have particular facial features that we are proud of. It may be the eyes, or the mouth; perhaps it's the whole face. With an attractively made up face, you can bring the focal point above your neck instead of leaving it lower down on that body part you want to camouflage.

Let's refer to your face—framed by your hair and your neckline—as your *Personality Center*.

The fashion portrait that shows you to the world must focus on your Personality Center, not your figure faults. To accentuate this area, you must take five things into consideration:

- Good makeup
- The right hairstyle for your face, neck and body
- The right neckline for your dresses, blouses, and sweaters
- The right shape and color of glasses for your face
- Creative accessories, such as scarves and jewelry

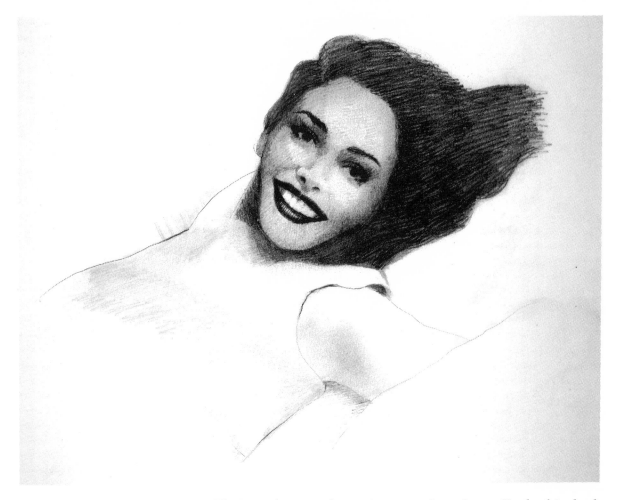

First you have to determine your face shape. To do this, look into a mirror and pull your hair back. Really look at the shape of your face. You will fit into one of the five shapes: oval, square, heart, round, long. To keep your Personality Center in harmony you must be careful not to duplicate the shape of your face with your hair, neckline, or jewelry. For example:

- A round face shouldn't wear round glasses
- A round face shouldn't wear a round necklace
- A round face shouldn't wear round necklines
- A round face can wear such items as square-framed

glasses, several long necklaces, or a V-neckline
- An oval face can wear anything; other shapes need to be careful

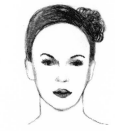

Long

Your hairstyle should not exaggerate the shape of your face. If your face is long and thin, you will want to add fullness to the sides to balance it. If your face is round or square, you should keep the hair away from the sides. The length of the hair is where the eye goes. There are many excellent books on determining the right hairstyle for your face. Better yet, when you see a hairstyle you like, ask what stylist cut it and get a free consultation from that person.

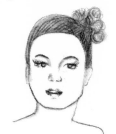

Square

MAKEUP

Ancient Egyptian beauties knew the value of makeup. They had mirrors, tweezers, eyeliner, and lotions just as we do today. Egyptian women of standing never left home without a beauty case filled with ivory combs and vials of perfumes and creams.

Roman ladies conditioned their skin with cool cucumber sticks and rose petal face packs. Some of the more potent face-saving mixtures contained unusual ingredients, like blood and crocodile excrement.

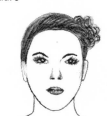

Oval

In the early 1600s, American colonists had to resort to home concoctions as beauty aids. Bacon was used to cover the face to soften the skin and delay wrinkles. Face powder consisted of egg shells ground up and mixed with water. Lips were reddened by sucking on lemon rind. Cheeks were pinched to bring out a rosy color.

Mascara wasn't introduced in America until Empress Eugenie brought some over in the later half of the nineteenth century. In 1887 zinc oxide was first used as a face powder. Innovative beauty aids quickly followed: oval tubes for lipsticks, powder boxes called "compacts," eye shadow, and facial packs of mud. Today, an amazing, sometimes confusing assortment of cosmetics is available to the beauty-minded woman.

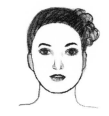

Round

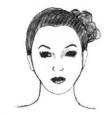

Heart

Today's cosmetic products do not have such bizarre ingredients (although we do smear our lips with petroleum products). Yet the concept of using cosmetics has not changed over the centuries—they are applied to enhance a woman's facial features. The word "cosmetics" comes from the Greek *kosmos,* meaning order and harmony. Yet too many women don't know how to apply makeup harmoniously.

Answer these questions:
- Do you use cosmetics?
- Do you use too much?
- Do you use too little?

Chances are you're using too little, especially at home, where brushing your teeth and running a comb through your hair frequently takes care of the morning's beauty routine. Oh, sure, you might slop on a little lipstick to sneak out of the house to pick up a quart of milk. Of course, that's the day you'll bump into your husband's ex-wife at the check stand, looking like she's on the way to a presidential inauguration.

Whether you work inside the home or outside, it's important to wear makeup. It makes you feel better and lets your true beauty shine through. Daytime makeup is a bit softer. For an evening on the town you'll just use a little more of everything. Makeup can make you come alive! Not just your face, but your whole personality. A little blush, eye shadow, and lipstick can bring out your eyes and add drama and excitement to your face.

It's hard to believe that only a relatively few years ago the use of makeup had a negative connotation, a leftover idea from the turn of the century, when anyone wearing lipstick was called "that hussy!" This new turn of the century says, "Cosmetics are in!"

What you must remember in buying cosmetics, regardless of price range, is that they all have virtually the same ingredients. Many cosmetic companies are supplied by outside laboratories. Some, such as Revlon, have their own labs. The only advantages that expensive cosmetics have over cheaper items are classier aromas and fancier containers. If you're paying top price for your makeup, you are paying for packaging and promotion.

I once asked a makeup consultant for a major cosmetic company if she really believed her line was superior to drugstore products. She replied haughtily, "It's the difference between driving a Cadillac and a Ford." Then she laughed. "Of course, they both get you there."

All product lines have some good products and some bad. If it makes you feel better to buy more expensive cosmetics and you think they work better for you, great. If it makes you feel like you're being ripped off when purchasing the pricey products, don't. Shop around, especially at drugstores or at-home sales instead of department stores. Let your pocketbook be your guide.

Unfortunately, at most drug stores there are no sample testers. Some do have samples locked away and will get them out if you ask. If you can't test it, don't buy it.

At-home sales companies are a good choice. You can test all you want in the comfort of your home, and the prices are less than department stores and a bit more than drugstores. Remember, if you buy a cosmetic you don't like or are allergic to, take it back along with the receipt. They will give you a refund.

What you must remember in buying cosmetics, regardless of price range, is that they all have virtually the same ingredients.

I have always been amazed by the changes that can take place on a woman's face with the proper use of cosmetics to enhance her features. The dramatic before-and-after photos in magazines and on television are positive proof of what makeup can do. I am fascinated by these makeovers and the visual transformation of a Plain Jane into a glamorous person. It's like having that fairy godmother wave a magic wand over Jane's face. The inherent beauty suddenly materializes.

Women are now free to be attractive, each in her unique way, and part of that look is makeup. A woman wears makeup; makeup does not wear the woman. Makeup doesn't hide, it enhances. Makeup should make you look and feel good.

Now that you have prepared your skin, let's try a makeup

makeover. If you're new at using makeup, practice when you have lots of time, not when you're hurrying to go to work or a special event. With a little practice you will be able to do your whole face in ten minutes, maximum. It takes only five minutes for a quick but acceptable job, fifteen minutes for a deluxe job.

Most women wouldn't wear clothes that are fifteen years old, yet they'll wear their makeup the same way for just as long. It's time for an update. Take advantage of home sales reps or department store makeup artists who will help you with your technique. Don't feel pressured to buy cosmetics that you don't want or need.

With a little practice you will be able to do your whole face in ten minutes, maximum.

Tools for Makeup

Far more important than how much you pay for cosmetics is what you put them on with: sponges and brushes. No professional makeup artist would think of using anything but the proper tools. Now's the time to invest in natural bristle brushes. They will last for years, if not a lifetime. Natural bristles have a cuticle (just like our hair), so powders will cling. Artificial brushes are slick and do not have any cuticle.

Have you ever bought a cheap paint brush and had the bristles come out while you're painting? You don't want that to happen to your face, so buy quality, either in a set or individual brushes. The key to good makeup is blending, and for that you need quality brushes.

Tools List

Mirror and Lighting I've been to mobile homes and mansions, both of which can have inadequate lighting in dressing rooms and bathrooms. The solution is a lighted makeup mirror. If your eyesight isn't what it used to be, use the magnifying side. If you don't have a vanity table to set the mirror on, hang it on the bathroom wall.

Cosmetic Sponges I prefer the triangular ones that can be purchased in a drugstore. The better quality ones can be washed and used many times. The lesser quality sponge begins to crumble after a few applications, so just throw it away.

Powder Brush This is used to apply loose powder and is your largest and most expensive brush.

Blush Brush Even when you buy an expensive blush, you only get a tiny brush. Throw that one in the garbage and buy a big brush so you can blend easily.

Small Eye Shadow Brush Use this to apply shadow in the eye creases.

Slant Brush Use to apply eye shadow to the lid for powder eyeliner and to smudge eyeliner lines.

Blending Brush Use to blend eye shadows after application.

Lipstick Brush Use to contour and shape lips and to blend lip liner pencil with lipstick.

Eyelash Curler This "medieval-looking" invention hasn't changed in fifty years. It curls your lashes.

Contour Brush This (optional) brush has a flat side to contour cheekbones without looking like you have a brown stripe down your face. If you don't do cheek contour, you won't need it.

PAINTING YOUR FACIAL CANVAS

Now that you have the tools, you are ready to begin applying the makeup.

Undercoats

Before you apply your regular foundation you may need a bit of special makeup for special problems. For instance, if your skin is sallow, try a pink or lavender undercoat before the foundation. Any major department store has a variety of colors of undercoats.

 Magic Trick

Here's a trick I call the "Halloween cover up." If you have a very ruddy complexion or tiny blood vessels near the skin surface, use a green undercoat on the red areas. Then blend. The green color will neutralize red. Great for pimples, age spots, blemishes too. Follow with foundation.

Foundation

This originated in Hollywood when makeup artists needed a skin covering that would photograph well under studio lights. Thick and greasy, the foundation resembled theatrical grease paint used by stage actors. There were very few colors to choose from, and it was impossible to match all the skin tones. That's where the concept of "wearing a mask" originated. The old foundations also caused skin problems.

The new formulas that have evolved offer a wonderful array of oil- or water-based foundations with colors to match every skin tone and look completely natural.

If you don't need any undercoating, your makeup routine can begin with foundation. It should be color-keyed to your skin tone: a rosy beige without pink if you have cool tones, a warm beige if you have golden tones, and a true beige if your skin is ruddy. The shade will be lighter or darker depending how fair or dark you are.

The color should match so well that you can blend it at the jawline (never onto the neck) and there will not be a noticeable color difference. You can't test a color on your wrist at the department store, because your wrist is not the same color as your face. Test a color at your jawline; even better test on your whole face in natural light. Wear the foundation home to see how long it lasts. If you can't test it, don't buy it. It is important that foundation does not look like a mask. You simply want to even out the skin, not cover it up. Too much foundation and you'll look "painted." Strive for a natural look.

Take a non-porous cosmetic sponge (never use your fingers) and blend the foundation on your face from your hairline to your jawline. That includes your lips and eyelids. The sponge helps you blend perfectly, even over large pores. For an even lighter touch, dampen the sponge and squeeze it dry, then apply the foundation.

When you work on your face, do it in upward strokes. Remember, gravity is pulling your skin down as you mature. There are only two times when you should work down your face. First, when you apply foundation, and second, when you apply powder. The reason is to make the facial hair lie down, not stand up.

Too much foundation and you'll look "painted." Strive for a natural look.

Concealer

Now it's time for a little concealer under your eyes to make those dark circles and valleys vanish. This is done on top of your foundation.

Lighter colors bring things forward, dark colors cause them to recede, so use a shade that is lighter than your foundation. Try one of the yellow concealers, which negate blue.

Apply and blend concealer with a small brush, blending under the eyes and close to the nose. If you put concealer under the whole eye, you might end up looking like a raccoon.

Powder

Use your largest brush to lightly dust a translucent loose (as opposed to pressed) powder (light, medium, or dark) over your face, eyes, and lips. Use downward strokes in the direction facial hairs grow.

Loose powder helps set your makeup, gives a light matte finish that hides wrinkles, and blots oily skin. Use a pressed compact powder only for touch-ups throughout the day, if necessary. Now the canvas is ready for the exciting part—color!

COLORING THE CANVAS

Eyes

The eyes take the most time and the most practice, but they are the focus of your face and personality. The eyes have been called "windows to the soul," so let's decorate those windows. There are dozens of ways to apply eye shadow. Trends come and go. Here is a method 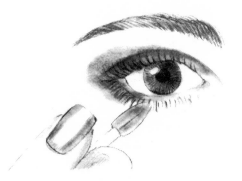 that works on almost all eyes; you can experiment with other ways.

Apply in three colors: light, medium, and dark. Using a sponge-tipped applicator or a shadow brush, apply the lightest (a nude, natural color or a very soft natural pink) over the entire lid, up to the brow. Brush the medium color into the crease of the eye, blending outward. Use the small slant-tipped brush to apply the darkest color, laying the shadow just above the lash toward the outer edge and under the eye for a short way (sort of a sideways V).

Always keep the lines moving toward the end and up. No wings though.

Cool tones (Summer and Winter) should use smoky blues (no bright blues, please), smoky blue-green, gray, smoky lavender and purple, and taupe eye shadow colors—all neutral colors. Winters can use stronger colors. Summers will use softer, more muted tones.

Warm tones (Spring and Autumn) should use brown, olive green, copper, and smoky blues (no bright blues, ever. Bright blues should be illegal!), or any color in the warm spectrum, all smoky neutral colors. Springs can use the stronger colors and Autumns the softer tones.

Cotton swabs are great erasers if you make a mistake.

Eyeliner

Use an eyeliner pencil in a neutral color (charcoal or black for cool, brown or taupe for warm) across the top of the lashes and underneath the bottom lashes a short way in. Blend and smudge with the slant brush. This also removes the wax that's in the liner so it won't move or run on your eye.

Light and shiny colors make the eyelids look plump. Dark and matte colors shrink them. If crepes are something you have around your eyes instead of something you eat, never use frosted eye shadow. Never. Use matte, instead. Always.

 Magic Trick

For a more defined line around your eyes, wet an eyeliner brush in water, dip it into a charcoal or brown eye shadow and use this as eyeliner. Blend with your slant brush so you can't see where the line begins or ends.

Eyebrows

Complete the framing of the eye by shaping the eyebrow. Eyebrows are ideally shaped as shown in the illustration.

Hold a pencil vertically beside your nose. Your brow should begin somewhere near the inside of your eye, as pictured.

Next, look straight ahead and hold a pencil to the outside of the iris. The arch, the highest part of the brow, should be there.

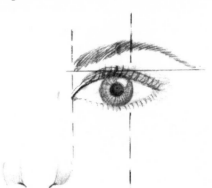

Then hold the pencil horizontally. The brow should end at the same level it began.

The brows should graduate in thickness gradually from thick to thinner, not *jump* from thick to thin. They shouldn't look like question marks above the eyes, or like you're always surprised.

If your brows are heavy, grow together, or need shaping you can tweeze. Never say "pluck." We pluck chickens. Tweeze brows. Be careful not to tweeze too much. Sometimes brows don't grow back. If fashion trends show very thin brows, ignore them. You don't want bald eyebrows later on.

Always tweeze from the bottom up, one row of hairs at a time. If you have long, unruly hairs, don't tweeze them out. Cut them shorter with cuticle scissors. It's always better for brows to be too full than too thin. Most people need to help nature and make some corrections with artificial brow color. Use a brow powder and a brow brush instead of a pencil. It will give you a totally natural look.

I have a friend who has no brows at all. She is able to look like she has them with a taupe-colored brow powder.

No one needs black brow powder or a pencil. Try brown,

charcoal, taupe, or gray. Be sure the brown isn't too red in tone. If you do choose a pencil, use small feathery strokes in the direction the hair grows, then brush through to blend.

Magic Trick

For an instant facelift, brows should be brushed straight up. To make them stay up, apply a brow gel or put a little hairspray on your brow brush and brush up.

Eyelashes

When using an eyelash curler, be sure the rubber pads are clean and in good condition. If the rubber is old, buy new refills. Always curl clean lashes before applying mascara so the curler won't stick to your lashes. Then apply mascara to upper and lower lashes. Several thin coats are better than one thick one. Use a brush to separate the lashes if they stick together. I find it easier to apply only one coat. No globs, please.

Cheeks

Don't color the apple of your cheeks unless you want to look like a circus clown. Hold three fingers up beside your nose; the last finger will be touching the highest part of your cheekbone. Begin blush there, working back toward the ear and hairline and up toward the eye. This will frame the eye and lift the face. Your blush should never be lower than your nostrils on your cheek.

Always use a large blush brush for perfect blending. Use less blush for day, more for evening. Cools should use blue-based colors, warms yellow-based colors.

Magic Trick

For cheekbones that give the face a slender contour, brush a darker blush just below the cheekbone. A soft brown blush is best. Apply with a special contouring brush so you can be sure it's blended perfectly.

Lips

"Speak softly and carry a big lipstick" is the rallying cry of the modern woman. To apply lipstick, use a lip fix if you need to control any bleeding of color. You've already powdered your lips, which helps the color last longer.

You should use a lip-liner pencil in a shade that will blend with your lipstick. Have you seen women walking around with a brown line around their lips? That's a no-no. Shape your lips just inside or outside the natural line if they need correction.

Most lips are asymmetrical, and it's impossible to even and shape them with a thick chunky tube of lipstick. No professional makeup artist would be caught without a lipstick brush to correct an imperfect mouth. So dip your brush in your color and blend your pencil line, and perfect your lip line. Then fill in the rest of your lips with the tube.

These steps take a little time, but your mouth outline will stay most of the day (that is, if you keep away from a greasy hamburger). You can touch up occasionally with your lipstick tube.

Magic Trick

For a pouty lower lip, blend a touch of light pink or white lipstick in the center of the lip.

After lips are finished, lightly hold a tissue over your mouth and apply powder gently with your powder brush on top of the tissue, over the lips. This will set your lipstick so it stays for hours without leaving lipstick kisses on coffee cups and glassware.

Cool tones can use all shades of pink lipstick, as well as rose, mauve, blue-red, true red, and wine. Warm tones can use all the shades of peach and true-red to orange, or copper-red and brown tones.

If the lipsticks you own are not the right color, throw them away. If you still have a tube of Tango Torment that you bought for the school prom (it looked great on the back of your hand), toss it out. I know, we are all great savers, and we hate to throw away anything in the cosmetic line. As Erma Bombeck once wrote, "If I threw away a tube of lipstick every day for the next three months, I would still have enough left over to write my phone number on 500 restroom walls. I refuse to discard my mistakes.... There's a shade called Bubble Gum Grape that matches a blouse that makes me look like I'm recovering from a malaria attack."

Voila! There you are.

You have drawn attention to your face with the right makeup application and taken it away from your figure flaws.

Just like magic.

If you still have a tube of Tango Torment lipstick that you bought for the school prom, toss it out.

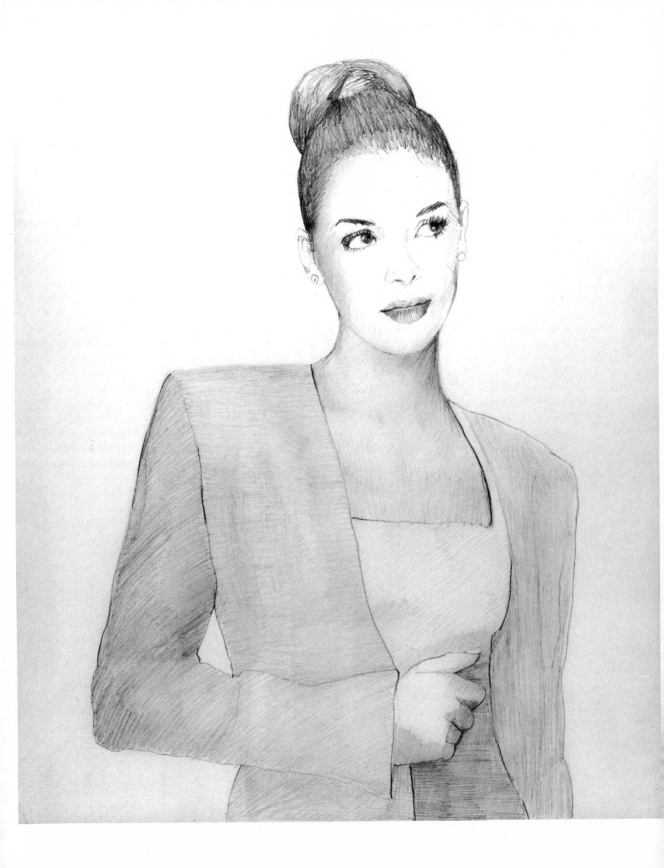

CHAPTER SEVEN

Silhouette Semantics

Creating an Illusion with Clothes

*"It's not who you are, it's what you wear.
I mean, who really cares
who you are?"*

—Anonymous

One day not too long ago I was scheduled to do a runway fashion show with a twenty-year-old model I had worked with several times before. She had it all: great figure, beautiful skin, lovely face. I thought she was one of the prettiest girls I had ever seen.

In the dressing room prior to the show, she started fussing with her nose, dabbing extra makeup on it, adding powder, then pushing it out of shape with her finger while cocking her head from one side to the other to see her profile in the mirror. Finally, she sighed, turned to me, and said, "I have an awful nose."

For the first time I really looked. She was right. She had a bad nose. It was too long, with a kink in the middle of the bridge. I had never noticed it before, and had she not pointed it out to me, I *never* would have noticed. Every time I saw her again I couldn't help but see her nose.

Another friend, well into her fifties, once said to a group of us, "I have the biggest head!" We all laughed. She blushed. "No, I'm not talking about ego; my head is too large for my body." I had known this woman for three years, and I had never noticed. But since she pointed it out, I looked. Now I always think of her as "the lady with the big head."

The best and cheapest way to camouflage your minuses is not to tell anyone about them. People are too busy worrying about their own; they'll never notice yours. Don't reveal those elephantine ears you have hidden so well under your hair, or that Romanesque nose that is a bit crooked, those stubby fingers, or thick thighs. If you just keep quiet, chances are no one will ever notice.

The best and cheapest

way to camouflage

your minuses is not

to tell anyone

about them.

That is, unless you flaunt your flaws by wearing the wrong clothes and colors or by applying garish makeup (or none at all) or by wearing your hair in a style that went out with hula hoops.

For instance, I know that my legs are a bit too large and I am too long-waisted; but I never tell anyone (until now, but that's all I'm going to tell!). I dress to correct those flaws by wearing the proper length skirt for my legs. (The hem comes above or below the widest part of the calf so it doesn't draw attention to that part of the leg.) I also wear slightly darker hose, which has a slimming effect. To keep my waist in proportion to the rest of my body, I wear wide belts, shorter jackets, or longer skirts.

I have a friend who is the best dressed, best made-up and best coifed woman I have ever met. Everything she wears is perfect. Her outfits look like they have been designed specifically for her. She has style. Yet if you look closely, her basic features are terribly unattractive, and her figure is much too angular. My husband refers to her face as being "horsy"—but he always adds, "a thoroughbred horse." Her features are indeed horsy: a long thin face with a jutting jaw and Roman nose. Her profile, the *silhouette* of her face, is unattractive. But with the right makeup and hairstyle, and clothes that accentuate her assets and the regal way she carries herself, she always creates the illusion of being an extremely attractive woman.

The trick is to enhance your figure assets and at the same time disguise your figure faults (let's call them figure "challenges"). With a little sleight of hand, a magical incantation or two, and some creative dressing, you can look better—instantly!

You do it with illusion.

SIMPLE ILLUSIONS

Certain geometric patterns create optical illusions. Remember this simple line drawing?

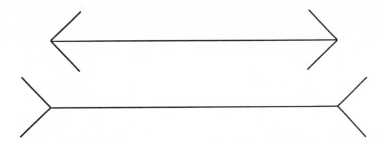

At first glance the top line appears shorter; but when measured it is the same length as the lower one. You want your optical illusion to instantly make you slimmer or wider, depending on your body. A similar illusion can be applied to these block figures.

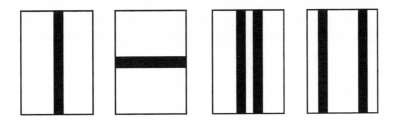

Vertical lines add to the apparent length. Placing vertical lines closer together heightens the illusion. The rectangle with the horizontal bar appears shorter than the figure with the single vertical bar. This simple illusion can easily be applied to clothes.

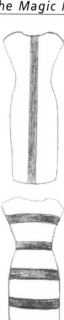

Vertical Straight Lines

The eye will follow a straight line faster and more directly than a curved line. That means that if you are short or a large size, vertical straight lines make you appear taller and slimmer. A vertical line in the center of the garment takes the eye away from the side bulges and makes you appear taller. Wraparound skirts also have vertical lines and are slimming.

Horizontal Lines

These lines emphasize width and are used if you want to look heavier, wider, or shorter. *They should never be worn by a larger person.* How many times have you seen someone with a protruding stomach wear a tight T-shirt with horizontal stripes? An unflattering combination.

Diagonal Lines

Lines that run diagonally from the shoulder of the dress to the waist, or even as far as the hem of the skirt, in one broad sweep create an illusion of slimness and movement. Diagonal lines can also mask poor figure proportions, such as slender shoulders and wide hips (the typical "pear" shape).

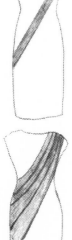

Curved Lines

These graceful, flowing lines are reminiscent of a Roman toga and effectively accent good features, such as the face. Figure assets can also be successfully highlighted or flaws camouflaged with curved lines.

These simple illusions are the basis for your trunk full of tricks. More magic is done with something called "silhouette semantics."

SILHOUETTE SEMANTICS

Etienne Silhouette (1709–1767) was a French finance minister with stingy habits. He objected to the high cost of portraits for officeholders in the government and proposed a cheaper form of likeness, a profile done in one solid color—black. Etienne's "silhouette" can be applied to today's body shape.

If you look carefully at an attractive woman's silhouette, you can find defects, such as a nose that's too big (Barbra Streisand), legs that are too stocky (Hillary Clinton), hips that are too wide (Hillary again), or a bust that's too small (Michelle Pfeiffer).

Cindy Crawford says she was called "Moleface" as a child. She was self-conscious about the mole on her upper lip until she appeared on the cover of Vogue. "I decided that if they liked it, it was okay," Cindy recalled. Movie star Geena Davis said she was an awkward, six-foot-tall teenager. "I never had dates in high school."

Actress Jane Seymour is extremely slender and small-busted, with a nose that is a bit too large for her heart-shaped face. Yet in person the eye is drawn to her smooth complexion, elegant carriage, and her fashionable attire. Seymour exudes beauty. The camera agrees. She says of herself, "I am definitely not the prettiest or most beautiful person in the world. There are many women who are more spectacular looking—but the camera does find things. I'm fortunate; I'm working with an instrument that loves me."

Everyone has flaws. Nobody's body is perfect.

Before we can drape those designer clothes on that newly aligned posture, it is necessary to discover your body assets and challenges. Let's start with the assets first.

ASSETS

We all have body parts, some we like, some we don't.

Everyone can produce a long list of parts they don't like, but in my "Magic Makeover" seminars I ask each person to name their favorite part. I always feel sorry when someone can't think of a single one. To give her confidence, I have the class point out the features they like about her.

Everyone has at least five good features. What are yours?

- Vibrant, glossy hair
- Fascinating eyes
- A lovely shaped mouth
- A beautiful complexion
- A well-proportioned body
- A great bosom
- Elegantly shaped legs
- Beautiful hands
- Pretty feet

How do you call attention to those features?

- With chic clothes
- Properly applied makeup
- The right hairstyle
- With accessories—jewelry, shoes, scarves, belts
- With color

Your answer to the second question should have been "All of the above." All of them can work together to draw attention to your outstanding assets.

Here are a few simple asset-enhancing tricks that can be done with clothes that will focus attention on your best features.

Face Eyes, hair, lips, or overall facial shape. Wear:
    Collars
    Turtlenecks (long neck)
    Cowls (short neck)
    Ruffles
    Scarves
    Jewelry—necklaces, earrings

Torso Balanced bustline, waist, and hips. Focus attention by wearing:
    Large brooches or pins
    Necklaces
    Wide belts
    Dresses with pockets
    Outfits with patterns
    Almost anything!

Legs Long and slender. Draw attention down by wearing:
    Sheer hose
    Slit skirts
    High-styled or colored shoes
    Sandals with no hose

Hands Wear:
    Nail polish
    Rings
    Bracelets

Enhancing your best features is important. A teenager walked into my classroom, a bewildered girl in baggy jeans, her face almost hidden by a massive hairdo. She was shy and sensitive and afraid to look at me. Her hair was a curtain draped between herself and the outside world. One night I pulled her hair back to show the class how it could be restyled. It was then I realized the girl had beautiful, expressive eyes. She was pretty. With her hair styled properly for her face, she gained confidence—and beauty. She went on to become one of the top fashion and swimsuit models in the country. Her name? Kathy Ireland.

BODY SHAPE

Take a good hard look to find out where your body challenges are, then do something about them.

Don't flaunt your flaws; camouflage them by emphasizing your assets. Before we start camouflaging, it is necessary to determine your body shape.

Your body shape is what you were born with, and it isn't predicated on how much you weigh. If you were born with small shoulders and large hips that give you the shape of an eggplant, then you can be a small eggplant, a medium eggplant, or a large eggplant. You will always be an eggplant, but you don't have to look like one. Simply pop in some shoulder pads to balance those hips.

Actress/singer Cher has a straight body shape, without much of a waistline. She knows how to highlight her assets, the well-proportioned legs and marvelous olive complexion. To show off her skin tone, Cher uses makeup well. To draw attention to her legs, she wears slit skirts. To camouflage her straight torso, she wears belts loosely below the waistline. One stroke of color adds to her height (which is only five-foot-five) and slims her waist.

If your hips are too big, then say to yourself that you are "hippy." If you are built more like a barrel than an hourglass, then admit it. Take a good hard look to find out where your body challenges are, then do something about them.

First, classify your body into one of these basic shapes.

- Balanced
- Hourglass
- Straight
- Inverted Triangle
- Triangle

Balanced

The balanced body shape and height is five-feet, five-inches to five-feet, nine-inches, with weight in proportion to bone structure. The hips and bust are close to equal, and the waist is ten to twelve inches smaller. Most off-the-rack clothing is designed with the balanced shape in mind. If you're lucky enough to have this body shape then your clothing selection will be relatively easy.

Do wear Fitted clothes
Clothes with horizontal lines or in two key colors
Vertical lines
Belts
Nearly anything

Avoid Overdressing

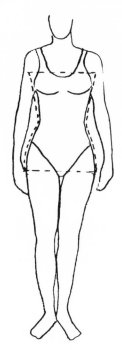

Hourglass

"Voluptuous," a la Dolly Parton or Elizabeth Taylor, defines this body shape. The full bust is equal to the full hip measurements, and the waist is small in proportion.

Do wear Necklines that promote a strong shoulder line
Chemises and tunics
Dresses
Longer skirts with vertical lines
A single stroke of color or monochromatic (different
tones of one color) color schemes
A looser waistline

Avoid Wide, tight belts
Tight sweaters
Skirts that are too short or too tight
Horizontal lines

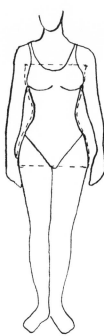

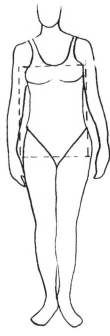

Straight

This body shape is in proportion from the shoulders to the hips, with little definable waistline.

Do wear Loose, flowing, semi-fitted clothes
One stroke of color or monochromatic color
One-piece dresses
A-line and wraparound skirts
Jackets below the waistline
Full-length coats with straight lines
Blouses or tunics
Belts that fall below the natural waistline

Avoid Belts, unless they are loose
Clothing made with heavy or bulky fabric
Blouses tucked into skirts
Anything tight at the waist
Anything that clings to the figure

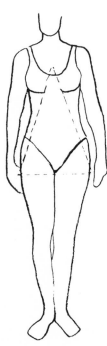

Triangle

This figure is generally referred to as "pear shaped." Weight is concentrated in hips and thighs wider than the shoulders.

Do wear Shoulder pads
A-line or flared skirts
Jackets with plenty of padding
Checks, prints, and light colors above the waist, darker colors below the waist
Large cowl necks and collars to broaden shoulders
Full-sleeve styles, such as dolman and raglan
Horizontal stripes above the waist with lines and detail that draw attention to the face
Narrow, matching belts

Avoid Wide skirts and narrow jackets
Drawing attention to the hips with a skirt in checks, prints, or light colors.

Unusual belts in contrasting colors
Clothing with small sleeves or narrow shoulders
Tight sweaters and blouses

Inverted Triangle

This body shape has broad shoulders and slim hips and may or may not have a large bustline.

Do wear Dark colors above the waist and lighter colors below
      the waist
Fuller skirts and slimmer blouses
Fitted, tailored jackets, not bulky ones
Pleated pants with fuller pants leg
Clothes with an A-line

Avoid Shoulder pads and breast pockets
Wide collars, frilly necklines
Blouses or dresses with ruffles
Puffed sleeves
Clingy tops

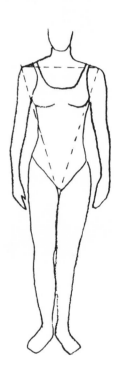

Tall or Petite

If you are very tall or quite petite, you need to complement your height with the following tips.

Tall—Five feet, nine inches or over

Do wear Wide belts and horizontal lines
Separates, such as jackets and skirts in contrasting
      colors
Large prints, checks, and plaids
Tunics, long suit jackets, three-quarter length coats,
      and lowered waistlines
Gathered or pleated skirts
Bulky sweaters, knit fabrics, loose-fitting coats and
      capes
Blouses and coats with full sleeves, wide cuffs

Large collars and scarves around the neckline
Large short jewelry, necklaces, and oversized bags

Avoid Clothing with vertical rows of buttons and trim
Long straight-line skirts or dresses
A slim-style dress that fits too tight
Vertical stripes or patterns
Anything small, such as jewelry and handbags
Short jackets
Empire lines

Petite—Five feet, four inches and under

Do wear Vertical lines in clothing
One stroke of color, or dress monochromatically
Vertical trims
A little longer skirt than current trends
Full-length coats with fitted or straight lines
Suit jackets that are fitted or do not fall more than six
    inches below the waist, like Chanel jackets
Prints and patterns that are small
Narrow belts
Empire waists
Handbags and jewelry to scale
Heels and wedgies instead of flats
Long necklaces

Avoid Big puffy sleeves and billowing skirts
Clothes with horizontal lines
Two starkly contrasting colors
Very short skirts
Heavy fabric
Massive jewelry, chokers, or short necklaces
Contrasting or wide belts and tight waists
Hats too large or overstuffed purses

Magic Trick
Petite isn't about width, it's about height. If you're 5'4"
or under you should shop in the petite departments.

Legs

If you want to slim your leg size:

Do wear   Dark hose
Boots
Straight-leg pants
Long skirts
Clothes that direct all interest above the waist
Tops that are light in color to draw the eye upward
Semi-fitted jackets
Simple shoes with low vamp and no horizontal straps
Shoes darker than your hemline

If you want to enlarge your leg size:

Do wear   Nude and lighter colored hose
Shoes with straps or any horizontal line
Boots
Long skirts
Lighter colored shoes, but no lighter than the hem line

Fingers

To slim thick fingers:

Do wear   Large rings
Nails in an oval shape
Large bracelets

Avoid Blunt or square-shaped nails

Necks

To lengthen a short neck:

Do wear Long necklaces
Necklines that are cowl, jewel, low, V, or mock turtle
Scarves lower on the neck

Avoid Turtlenecks
Choker or short necklaces

Waists

To lengthen short waists:

Do wear Belts the same color as your top
Belts that are not more than an inch and a half wide
over blouses
Chain belts that fall below the waistline

Avoid Wide belts the color of your skirt

Think about your good and bad points while you're shopping. Blend the right clothes with your body to make a coordinated whole. Think of yourself as a magician. Use line, texture, color, and design to create a picture of beauty.

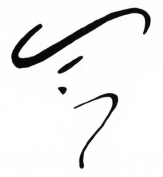

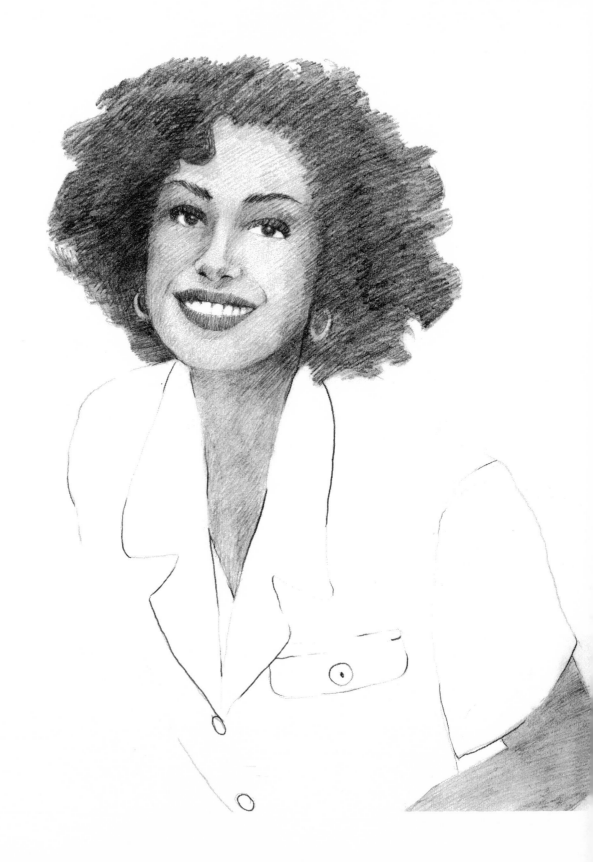

CHAPTER EIGHT

Style and Lifestyle

Discovering the Style that Fits You

"If fashion is punk rock, then style is an opera
(sung in Italian, of course):
one fleeting, one enduring."

—*Anonymous*

Why are you spending all that money just to buy your chorus girls *silk* lingerie?" the producer stammered to Flo Ziegfeld.

Ziegfeld leaned back in his leather chair and looked around his office. The walls were filled with huge framed photographs of beautiful women in flamboyant feathered headdresses and sequined show costumes. The producer persisted, "Silk underwear? It's too expensive! Besides, the audience never sees it under those costumes."

Ziegfeld answered with a smile. "Ah, but the girls know they have it on."

Ziegfeld understood that looking great also meant feeling great.

If you don't *feel* good in your clothes, if you don't love your clothes, chances are they aren't "you." If you have style, it will shift the focus away from your flaws. People will say, "That woman has style!" Remember the last time someone complimented you, said how great you looked? It gave your ego a lift.

Why did you look so good?

How did that outfit complement your figure?

What did it disguise?

What feature did it emphasize?

What color was it?

And finally, why was it the right style for you?

Ah...style. *What is style?*

STYLE

The dictionary defines style as the "current, fashionable way of dressing." That's an oversimplification. Style is how you express yourself through clothing with excellence, originality, and distinction.

Style is a quality of imagination and individuality expressed in one's actions and tastes. If you have "style," you know how to take a new trend or a new fashion and personalize it to make it work for you or skip it altogether if it's not right. *Style cannot be bought.* Style you create, fashion you buy. Style is not buying an exclusive designer gown for $2,000, but looking as though you have. Style isn't tangible. It's a sense of fun.

Style can be learned.

Some women are born with it, but they are few. Others acquire it with a little study, while others develop it through hard work.

I know a wonderfully stylish woman. She is a secretary in a large office and makes just enough money to survive. She is always dressed with flair. She has style. Yet she doesn't have a large wardrobe. As a matter of fact, every garment she owns fits in a tiny three-foot closet.

Style is deciding who you are and perpetuating it. *Fashion—* or fad—is a way of not deciding who you are. Fad is an isolated style that fades quickly. *Trends* affect many items and are wearable by many. Use trends in your wardrobe, not fads. Marching to someone else's drum can cost you thousands of dollars every season.

Each year the fashion industry decrees exactly what is "in style." They produce magnificent designs to show the eagerly waiting world. Fashion magazines run hundreds of color pages showing what's new, fashionable, and unique for the current season. They happily trumpet what the designers have crafted—just for you!

But maybe it's not for you.

Even if a designer could come up with a style that looked perfect on everyone's body, some people would look better than others. You see, *some women know how to wear clothes*—others just put them on.

Not everyone has inherent good taste. Some people look…well, not all together. They may look garish or cheap, unkempt or sloppy. Bad taste can be changed, but a person has to recognize she has it.

I knew two sisters, both in their mid-twenties, physically similar, who were at opposite ends of the spectrum when it came to dressing with style. One always looked sleek and smart—the other always looked like a pile of rumpled clothing. The problem was that the second sister didn't realize it. She *thought* she looked great.

One day, in frustration, the stylish sister said, "Okay, if you think you look so good, let's change clothes. You put on what I have on, and I'll get into your outfit."

It was a revelation. Like magic, their images were reversed. The styleless sister exclaimed wide-eyed, "You look awful in my clothes!" Then she looked at herself in the mirror and said, "Is that me? I look great."

Some women seem to sense when a garment is exactly right for them and shows off their assets to the best advantage. They seem to be born with a scarf-tying gene, one that knows the right way to accent a new suit, when to add a belt, how to turn up a collar, or how to mix a wild assortment of color and have it all look smashing.

They have style.

You can develop your own personal style.

Can you acquire chic?

Sure.

Taste is a product of your background.

Good taste can be learned.

Just because you learn your own style doesn't mean you never have to change again. Style is consistency tempered with growth. Women who don't change, age themselves.

DEVELOPING YOUR OWN STYLE

First, buy or borrow all the fashion magazines and catalogues you can get your hands on. Raid the newsstands. Take the magazines to the comfort of your living room and study them. Absorb what you are seeing on each page. Pore over the fashion advertisements and the editorial layouts. Try to figure out why the model in the picture looks so good in that outfit.

Then look again. You can't comprehend it all at once. Look at the accessories. Then look at the hairstyles, the models' makeup.

After studying some of the pictures you will tell yourself, "I wouldn't be caught dead in that!" Look at the picture again and ask yourself a better question, "How can I ever wear that?" Perhaps you can't. Perhaps it *is* all wrong for you. By studying every picture you will soon be able to recognize what is good and bad for your body. *Make a game of it.* Ask yourself these questions about each picture:

- Would I look good in that outfit?
- Is it right for my body shape?
- Is it in my color?
- Will it emphasize my assets?
- Can it camouflage any flaws?
- How could I add flair to it? A new belt? Tie on a scarf? Different shoes? Bigger handbag? Hat?

Do this "look and see" exercise over and over again—picture after picture. You can do it! It's like learning a craft, a craft that enables you to recognize ways to make clothes look good on you. You will be able to feel what the designer is doing and how he accomplished the design. (Most designers had to learn their crafts too. They weren't born geniuses. Few of them were born in Parisian designers' trunks. Ralph Lauren and Calvin Klein were born in Brooklyn.)

Even if you don't like the designs you see in a magazine, at least try to understand the trends and the latest fashion colors. Realize what's going on from an objective viewpoint, not an emotional one. You will soon know you don't have to buy a new wardrobe every year to look trendy. You can upgrade by simply buying a few new accessories. Perhaps all you need is a new pair of shoes, or a belt or a purse to add to your basic classic clothes. You can always buy a blouse or a scarf in this year's "in" colors if it flatters your skin.

 Magic Trick

Take that old A-line that has been hanging in the closet and experiment with it. Spice it up with a fashionable new scarf or belt and—*presto!* Like magic you will have an up-to-date outfit. (It will also save you a lot of money.)

You can begin to build ideas for your basic wardrobe on these ideas, ones that will suit you—and your lifestyle.

Determining Your Lifestyle

There are four basic lifestyle classifications that determine the majority of the clothes you have in your closet. They are:

Homemaker

Career (or professional)

Socially active

Combination of the above

Most of your fashion budget should be spent on clothes that suit the major portion of your lifestyle. That means you don't have to dress like a Ford pickup truck because you are home most of the day. Perhaps a Chevrolet wardrobe would fit you better, or even a Jaguar. You don't have to look like a graduate from the Phyllis Diller school of charm just because you're a stay-at-home mom raising a family. You need to look good and feel great every day.

Too many women think they should spend most of their money on a special "dress-up" wardrobe that they rarely wear. A closet should not look like it belongs to Sharon Stone if you don't share her lifestyle. It is much better to buy one simple elegant evening gown that will stay in style, or, better yet, separates that can be changed easily, such as evening pants or a long skirt with different tops. A good quality outfit is a better value in the long run.

If you are a **homemaker** you don't need many dressy daytime clothes; rather, a practical but smart wardrobe to wear around the house is called for. You can buy fun sports outfits in an array of shorts, pants, slacks, and sweatsuits.

If you are a **career** person and work outside the home full time, then you should spend the most on dressing professionally, and less on casual clothes.

If you're **socially active**, you must emphasize daytime dresses and suits, cocktail and evening clothes, with fewer casual items.

Some women work part time and will need a **combination** wardrobe that will cover all three lifestyles.

Let your basic lifestyle clothes dominate your wardrobe. But no matter what that is, it is also necessary to determine your personal "fashion style."

You don't have to dress like a Ford pickup truck because you are home most of the day.

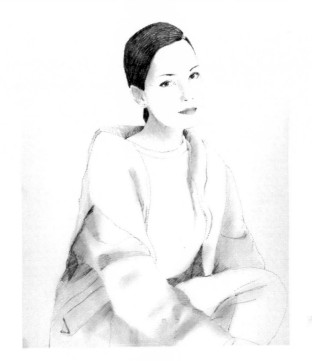

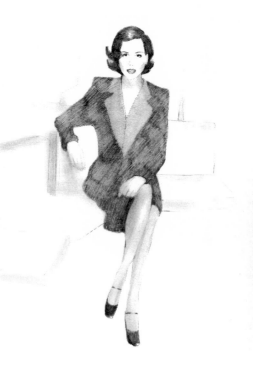

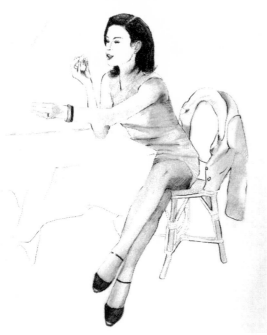

Homemaker

Career

Socially Active

Fashion Style

Your "fashion style" represents a range of attitudes in the way you prefer to dress for all occasions. These styles fit into four categories:

- Classic
- Avant-garde
- Romantic
- Country Casual

To determine which category fits you, take the following quiz. Of the four answers in each category, circle the one (or ones) that most closely show your taste in clothing.

FASHION STYLE QUIZ

1. **My favorite eveningwear is**
   A. Suit
   B. Evening pants or jumpsuit
   C. Dress
   D. Slacks and blouse

2. **My favorite daytime style is**
   A. Tailored suit
   B. Pants & boots
      worn with a cape
   C. Pastel print dress
   D. Jeans or cords with
      blouse or T-shirt

3. **My favorite colors are**
   A. Neutrals and solids
   B. Bold prints and
      bright contrasts
   C. Florals and pastels
   D. Bright colors in checks,
      stripes, and plaids

4. **My favorite coat is**
   A. Belted wraparound coat
   B. Fleece-lined jacket
   C. Shawl
   D. All-weather raincoat

5. **My favorite shirt is**
   A. Tailored silk blouse
   B. Heavily padded
      oversize blouse
   C. Ruffled blouse
   D. Cotton shirt

6. **My favorite fabrics are**
   A. Cotton, silk, wool, linen
   B. Metallics, ethnic prints,
      velvet, beaded
   C. Sequined, jersey, voile
   D. Denim, corduroy, blends

7. **My favorite accessories are**
   A. Fine jewelry
   B. Fad or ethnic jewelry
   C. Cameos, pearls, antiques
   D. Costume jewelry

8. **My favorite handbag is**
   A. Quality leather bag
   B. Firm constructed bag
      with handles
   C. Cloth or soft leather bag
   D. Canvas tote bag

9. **My favorite shoe is**
   A. Pump
   B. High-heeled boot
   C. Sandal
   D. Tennis shoe or flat boot

Total up your answers:

Total A's _3_ or 4

Total B's _____

Total C's _____

Total D's _____

If you totaled up more A's you fit into a Classic fashion style. B's, Avant-garde. C's Romantic. D's Country Causal.

Although the answers will indicate your basic style, you didn't fail if you had marks in several different categories. Most of us tend to be a combination of two or even three different styles, but one is predominant. When you're dressing, it's fine to combine two styles (Romantic, Classic, etc.), but don't combine three at one time. You'll look too convoluted.

 Magic Trick

Tear sheets: When you see an illustration you really like in a magazine, rip it out and put it in an envelope. Keep doing this for a month or so, then take the pictures out and see what you have. You will be amazed. For the most part they will be in one or two styles, either Classic, Romantic, Avant-garde, or Country Casual. That is your Style.

On the following pages are tips on what you should wear for each fashion style.

The **Classic** woman buys simple designs, such as tailored separates, that are in style year after year. A blazer and a plain skirt or pants will look good for a long time. She prefers solids over prints in major purchases because they are more flexible. She uses prints (if at all) in blouses and scarves. Her wardrobe dollar is spent on quality, not quantity. Typical fabrics for the classic style are natural ones, such as wool, silk, cotton, and linen. She also likes quality jewelry in classic designs. She knows that even classics change style approximately every seven years.

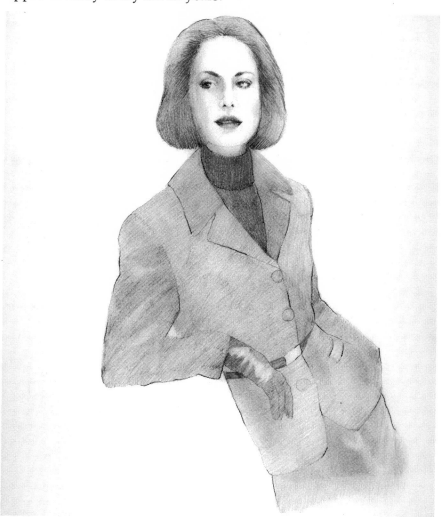

Classic

The **Avant-garde** styled woman dresses by following the latest fads, using ethnic styles, or even wearing costume-like outfits. She likes bright, bold fabrics and wild prints. She combines textures and designs in sometimes bizarre but fun and fascinating ways. Extremes are her thing. She loves large pieces of costume jewelry and isn't afraid to combine them with fine jewelry. She has a talent for discovering her own unique style. She has *panache*.

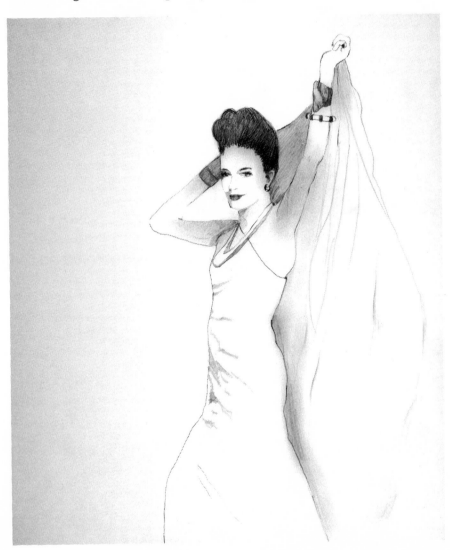

Avant-garde

The **Romantic** woman likes ruffles, soft-flowing fabrics, draping, and lace. She prefers dresses or skirts to pants. Her sweaters might be Angora. She likes rather small prints, such as pastel florals. She'll choose very feminine fabrics like velvet, lace, voile, rayon, and jersey or blends and cotton for casual wear. She likes delicate shoes or sandals rather than pumps. She will accessorize with flowers and ribbons. Her jewelry is more open and dainty than massive and heavy.

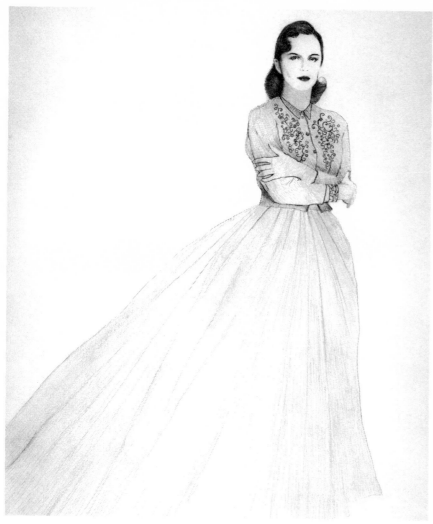

Romantic

Separates are the key to the **Country Casual**-styled woman's wardrobe. Her patterns and prints will be simple, but her fabrics will be bulkier and textured. Materials she'll use are wool, wool blends, denim, cotton, linen, corduroy, leather, knits, suede, and ultrasuede. Comfort is of primary importance. She prefers costume jewelry over real gold or silver accessories.

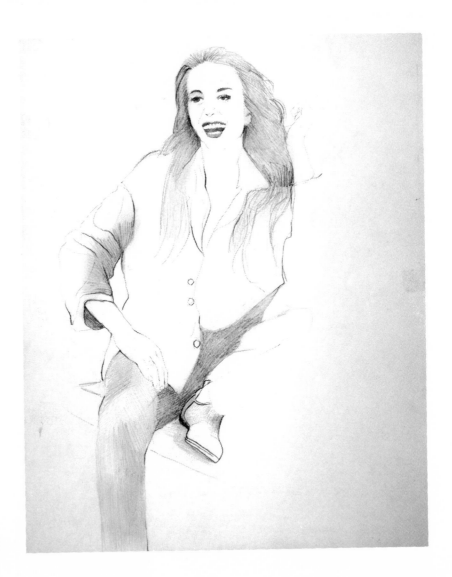

Country Casual

Don't forget, your hairstyle should go with your dominant style—classic hair for classic and casual looks. Romantic hair with romantic looks.

Watches should follow the style. You don't wear a sporty day watch with a cocktail dress. Just don't wear any at all if it doesn't blend with your outfit.

Nails can be classic or dramatic, depending on how they're manicured. Eyeglasses, too. Keep things blended.

One word of caution: A lifestyle makeover must evolve, not be an upheaval.

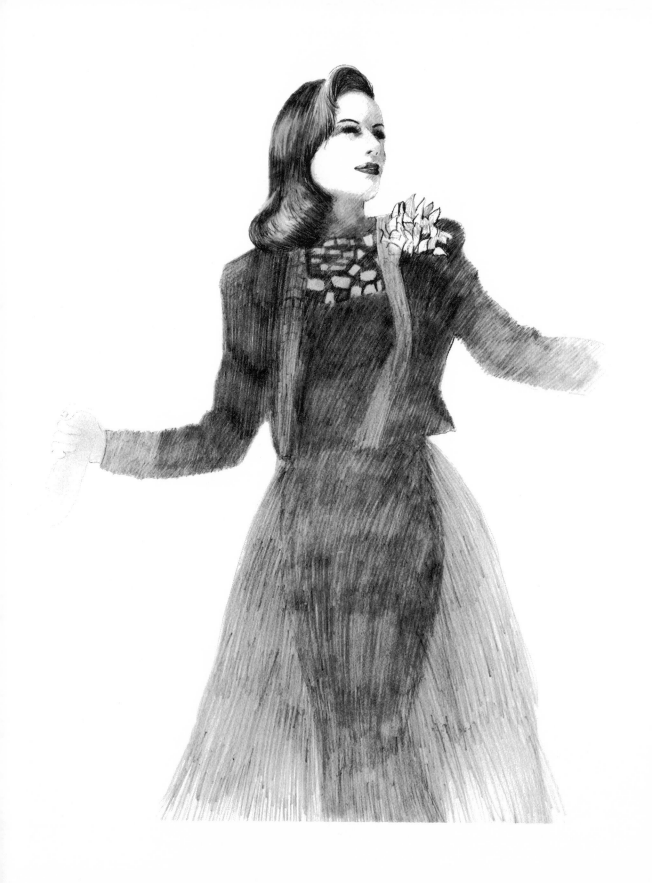

CHAPTER NINE

Fashion and Figures

What Fashion Can Do for Your Shape

*"Fashion is that thing which is soon
out of fashion."*

—Coco Chanel

In my grandmother's house hung a framed picture of my great-aunt, Zula Zong. Zula was not an exotic dancer or a snake charmer as her name seems to imply. She was a schoolteacher in the early 1900s.

Unlike her sister "school marms," she was always fashionably dressed, elegantly attired in the latest hats and the smartest lace blouses. She was so exceptional, she was selected by a magazine to pose for pictures illustrating how a schoolteacher could dress in the latest style.

As a child I used to stare at Zula Zong's photograph, thinking how wonderful she looked. (I also fantasized about how great it would be to have my picture in a magazine, a dream I kept alive through a marriage and two children until I took my first fashion modeling course at the age of forty.)

As I became fashion conscious, I came to realize that my great aunt looked elegant because the "high" fashions of her day were perfect for her figure. She had a round face, short stature, and her figure was hippy. The fashionable hats she wore (which looked like flying saucers) balanced her face and added height to her frame. The puffed-sleeve blouses also added to her bustline, and the floor-length dresses minimized her hips and made her look taller.

She was lucky. She was an hourglass woman in an era of hourglass figures. Fashion designers seemed to be styling their latest creations just for her. We should be so lucky.

Unfortunately, few fashion designers create something that is just right for your figure. At times it would appear they try to create clothes that no one could wear. Too often, as the fashion trends are paraded in the major design houses, women are heard to lament, "Who would wear that?" When the designers get too silly and the fashions too off-the-wall, it's time to jump ship. If the fashion makes you look ridiculous, don't wear it.

Too often designers create a fantasyland of fashionable excess. Are they really serious about having *every* woman in the world wear their styles? If that's true, then all women would have to have popped out of the same mold. Everyone would have to look like a mannequin, skinny all the way to the bone. Designers design their clothes to hang on human clotheshangers, not on the average woman's body. Not everyone is tall, thin, flat, and fair. In fact, only about 4 percent fit that mannequin mold. It's the rest of us who are normal!

Face it, the fashion figure you see in magazine illustrations is not attainable. Like the old drawings of pin-up calendar girls by Vargas, the body proportions shown in sketches in fashion magazines are wildly exaggerated. Fashion illustrators create a design abstraction that emphasizes the appealing lines of a garment. You are not going to look like that in it, nor would you want to. If you saw one of those drawings step off the page and walk down the street, you would think the city had been invaded by Martians.

In the eighties the layered look and loose-fitting clothes and tennis shoes came into vogue. The late Erma Bombeck observed a bag lady who was pawing through a trash can and noted that the street woman was wearing a plaid blouse, green sweater, mauve

You don't have to be tall, thin, flat, and fair to look good.

vest, and tan coat with a blue scarf over an oversized skirt that stopped just an inch above a pair of baggy socks and tennis shoes.

Bombeck wrote: "With the exception of the blue scarf and the plaid blouse, we were dressed alike." Bombeck went on to say, "It's hard to admit that style-wise bag ladies were twenty years ahead of their time. If someone had told me that I'd be walking around Manhattan in a pair of gym shoes wearing a skirt with more wrinkles than my grandmother, I would have laughed myself to death."

Sometimes the designers simply miscue. Do you remember the sack dress? It was fine for expectant mothers. The balloon-shaped design made everyone look pregnant, including the fashion models. In this rare case, the consumer recognized how unflattering the design was and rejected it. Unfortunately, the fashion industry has too often been able to dictate what all women must wear.

The most glaring example of one designer's ability to impose his personal will upon the female population was in 1947, when Christian Dior plummeted skirt lengths to everyone's ankles. The "New Look" was the single greatest coup in modern fashion history. Fellow designers oohed and aaahed in jealous appreciation, then copied the design for their own lines. With new sales forthcoming (after all, no woman had enough material to let down the hem of knee-length skirts), textile manufacturers went on buying junkets, dress shops greased up their cash registers, and department stores hired extra sales clerks.

The New Look was certainly new; but it was far from the right style for many women's body shapes. The expanse of material that drifted from waist to ankle made a woman look like a schooner under full sail. A short woman in the new-length dress looked like a sidewalk windup doll.

Over the next twenty years skirt lengths slowly inched higher, then suddenly (much to the chagrin of the designers) the miniskirt craze materialized. Confused, the designers argued among themselves about skirt lengths: some wanted them dropped to the floor again, others went faddish and designed micro-minis and hot pants.

The New Look was certainly new; but it was far from the right style for many women's body shapes.

The major catalogue houses, such as Sears and Montgomery Ward, were in a quandary. I remember looking through a catalogue to check out the new skirt lengths—only to discover there weren't any! Unable to determine the fashionable length, the companies copped out. The catalogue photos were all cropped above the models' knees.

The 1970s became known as the decade in which the delicate glass of high fashion was shattered. Women who wanted to be well dressed had to tiptoe through fragments of style, trying to find skirt lengths that felt comfortable and hemlines that naturally flattered the figure. Once the dust settled, it was obvious that there were no rules left. Anything was possible—minis, maxies, and micros. This legacy has held over into this decade. Today's woman can create her own successful fashion image, one that is correct for her lifestyle—and figure.

The 1970s became known as the decade in which the delicate glass of high fashion was shattered.

In an effort to discover designs that correspond to earlier ideas of grace and good taste, of flair and finesse, women have turned to such designers as Dana Buckman, Ellen Tracy, Giorgio Armani, all of whom consistently design flattering clothes.

I was recently introduced to Luis Estevez, the designer of my "favorite ever" dress from the early sixties. This elegant wool jersey dress was both backless and sleeveless, a dress that would be in style today. Estevez is still designing clothes, timeless classics in good taste. (I even had the good fortune to model at his grand opening in Santa Barbara, which showed his new line.)

Each year some designers create styles that are unusual or outlandish. Each season we hear that hems are up or down, shoulders are padded or bare, or waistlines are this or that. Why do we listen? How can anybody with a kindergarten education pay serious attention to these creative ramblings? The answer is simple—we like it. After all—whether we understand it or not—fashion is fun.

HOW TO STAY FASHIONABLE

Have you ever looked at a mature, *un*fashionable woman and been able to tell the year she got married? It's easy. That woman hasn't changed one thing about herself since the day she walked down the aisle twenty-five years ago. She's still wearing: a stiff bouffant hairdo, frosted pale lipstick, black liquid eyeliner (maybe even false eyelashes), and a dress design that went out of style about the same time the twist was becoming a dance craze.

True, that woman may think she has her own style, but instead her message to others is that she's totally behind the times. I know a very well-to-do lady, let's call her Amelia, who buys expensive designer gowns that flatter her rather abundant figure, and from the neck down she looks terrific. Unfortunately Amelia's hair looks like a pile of bleached straw, and she insists on wearing the same shade of frosted orange lipstick that she's worn for two decades. Not only is the lipstick color passé, it is also wrong for her skin tone. And it doesn't complement her beautiful clothes. From the neck up Amelia needs to be restyled.

Unless you want to look like you live in a time warp, changes must be made if you are to stay fashionable.

You may love your hairstyle. It's taken you many years to develop just the right thing that is flattering to your face shape and suits your lifestyle. That's great. But a few subtle changes are needed to keep it updated. You may also like the way you apply your makeup—the simple classic way. But unless you want to look like you live in a time warp (like Amelia), changes must be made to follow eye makeup trends and fashion lip colors.

How do you stay in style?

Easy: by reading the fashion magazines that I suggested, and determining which of the fashion trends are good for you and which ones to avoid. Remember, many avant-garde styles won't look good on problem figures. Look for modified versions of the new style. For each radical design there will be a toned-down version, one less extreme but still up to date.

Magic Trick
Attend a fashion show at your local department store.
That's where you'll see the modified versions. Check
out what's new and see if there is anything that's right
for you.

If you are on a limited budget, don't invest large sums on fad items. If you just *have* to have it, then buy an inexpensive version. When it's out of style next year, you won't mind tossing it.

It is best to make major purchases in classic styles and the basic colors that are right for you. You can add the year's fashion colors by wisely investing in a blouse, T-shirt, sweater, belt, scarf, shoes, or jewelry. These reasonably priced and versatile items can be mixed and matched to update your wardrobe.

But to have fashion work for us, we must discover how it can complement our natural figure proportions.

This can be done through what designers call the "fashion line."

THE FASHION LINE

The "line" of a garment is what the eye naturally follows when looking at an outfit. Why not use this natural line to influence what the viewer sees? Quite simply: if you want to appear taller and slimmer, you need an outfit with long continuous lines that draw the eye all the way from your neck to your toes.

Avoid styles that don't put you at the peak of your potential. Here's how to make the standard "fashion lines" work for you:

Triangle The emphasis is at the hemline with a narrower waist and slimmer shoulders. The design is excellent for melting away a large bustline.

Hourglass Shoulder and hemline emphasis is equal with the waistline accented. The fashion line works with the well-proportioned figure.

Inverted Triangle Emphasis is above the bustline, with a slim hipline. This design is for the large-hipped person.

Straight or Column The shoulder and hemline width are about the same. This is an excellent line for thick-waisted women.

Oval This line is characterized by equal balance from shoulder to hemline, with a slight emphasis on the waist. A great line for any figure proportion.

Diamond Shoulder and hemline are much narrower than the midsection of the design. Very good for thick waists.

Magic Trick

Analyze what the major fashion line is for the new season, then determine how it can be used to camouflage your figure challenges. Don't be afraid to disregard a fashion line if it is completely wrong for your shape. For instance, what if the fashion dictates oversize jackets and tops with slim pants? If you have narrow shoulders and large hips, you should be ecstatic. But if you're already top heavy, you will want to reconsider buying an expensive outfit that will make you look like a tank. Remember, you wear the clothes; don't let the clothes wear you.

To determine the most flattering styles of skirts, blouses, jackets, and pants, study the following drawings. Understand what figure faults they disguise—or accentuate.

Skirts

These are the classic styles that designers use in their fashion lines. Circle the ones that are complementary to your body shape.

1. **Straight skirt** Slender women only. Keep away if you're overweight. Emphasizes large hips.
2. **A-line skirt** Excellent for camouflaging large hips. Hangs away from the heaviest part of the hip. Flattering for all shapes.

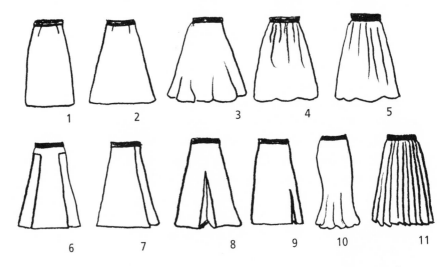

3. **Full skirt** In soft fabrics, it's one of the greatest styles for a full figure.
4. **Gathered dirndl** Excellent cover-up for the tummy.
5. **Gathered skirt** With all its fabric, it looks better on a slim hipline.
6. **Gored skirt** This style creates an illusion that leads the eye upward. Great for camouflaging large bottoms or hips.
7. **Wrap-around skirt** Good for larger hips. The focus is on a bold vertical line and not the hips.
8. **Center front pleat** Gives the same illusion as the wrap-around skirt. Makes you look taller and slimmer.
9. **Slit skirt** Slims large legs, makes short legs longer.
10. **Trumpet** Very hip-slimming.
11. **Pleated** Creates vertical lines. Good for large hips.

Jackets

1. **Single-breasted blazer** The classic standard. Flattering to the large-busted or short woman and to nearly everyone else.
2. **Double-breasted blazer** Be careful. Emphasizes a large bust. Flattering to tall, slim women.
3. **Hacking jacket** Large hips keep away from this design. Good for small-busted women.
4. **Chanel jacket** This style slims large hips and large busts. Also good for short women.
5. **Cardigan** Slims hips and is flattering to the large-busted. Good for short or full figure.
6. **Safari jacket** Good for most shapes. Avoid large upper pockets if you are big busted.
7. **Bolero** Great for small bustlines. Very bad for large bottoms.

Jacket sleeves should come to the bone at the base of the hand just below the wrist.

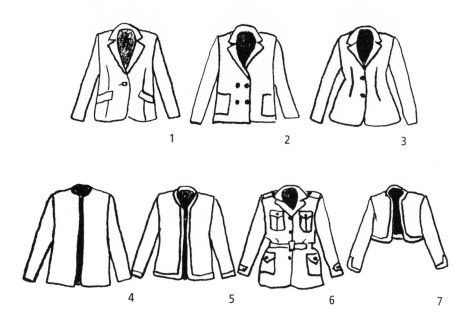

1   2   3

4   5   6   7

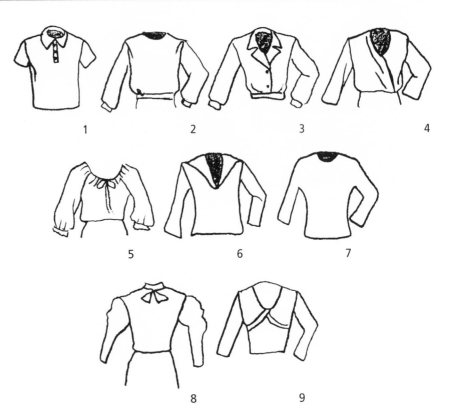

Blouses

1. **Polo shirt** Best worn by a woman with a slim to average figure. Be sure it fits loosely.
2. **Suit shirt** Great for all figure types.
3. **Shirtwaist** Flatters all shapes.
4. **Surplice** Has strong vertical lines that are good for all upper-body shapes.
5. **Peasant** Slim to average upper-body shape.
6. **Middy** Good for everyone.
7. **Long torso** Works for slim, average, and thick waists.
8. **Gibson** Okay for hourglass and slim figures.
9. **Empire** Excellent for most shapes.

Sleeves

1. **Sleeveless** Only good for a firm arm (without "cottage cheese" skin).
2. **Long-fitted sleeve** Good for thin arms and older ones.
3. **Short set-in** To be avoided if you have heavy upper arms.
4. **Short puffed sleeve** Good for average to thin arms.
5. **Dolman** Great for heavy upper arms, broad shoulders, and full figure.
6. **Raglan** Good for broad shoulders and heavy arms.
7. **Set-in tailored cuff** Good for heavy arms.
8. **Bell** Also flattering for heavy arms.
9. **Bishop** Really camouflages heavy arms.
10. **Angel** Good for everyone (except large busts).

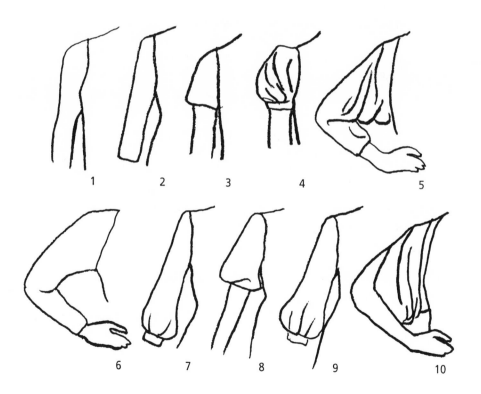

Necklines and Collars

In choosing necklines, do not repeat lines that are similar to your face shape. No round collars with round faces, or low V's with long faces. The size of the neckline should be balanced with the size of your figure, head, and length of your neck.

1. **Round (or jewel) neckline** Good for most necks.
2. **U-neckline** Makes the neck and face appear wider. Not recommended for a round face. Okay for large-busted and short neck.
3. **V-neckline** Good for a round face because it makes the neck and head appear longer. Also good for a large bust.
4. **Square neckline** Square faces keep away! A narrow face is widened.
5. **Bateau neckline** Shortens and widens face.
6. **Shawl collar** Lengthens a short neck and widens the shoulders. Good for a straight figure.
7. **Turtleneck** Does terrible things to double chins and short necks. Widens the face. Excellent for long necks (wrinkled necks, too). Aids a small bust.
8. **Peter Pan collar** Shortens and widens the face. Good for petite figures.
9. **Bow neckline** Like adding a scarf, this flatters the face. Because it is rather old-fashioned, wrap the ties around the neck instead of into a bow.
10. **Mandarin collar** Flattering for a long neck.
11. **Notched** Similar to V neckline. Good for round face and short neck.
12. **Halter** Needs broad shoulders and firm arms.

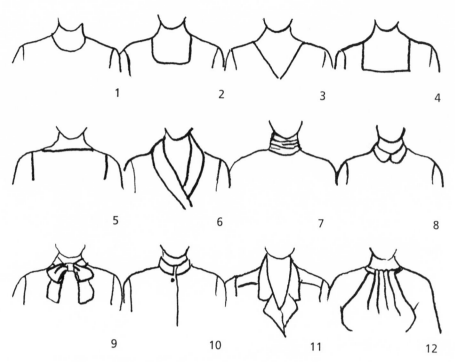

Shorts and Pants

1. **Short shorts** Thin to average legs look best in this style. Makes legs look longer.
2. **Bermuda** Best style shorts for heavy legs. Wear them a little shorter if your legs are short.
3. **Culottes** Good for all legs. Vary length depending on whether your legs are short or long.
4. **Straight-leg trouser** Flattering to every leg.
5. **Jeans** Loose style for heavy legs; tighter western leg for thin to average shape.
6. **Skinny-leg pants** Thin to average legs and hips only.
7. **Pajama leg** Good for most legs.
8. **Flare (or bell)** Great for all legs.

Realize that any pant leg that tapers in at the bottom makes the hips look larger.

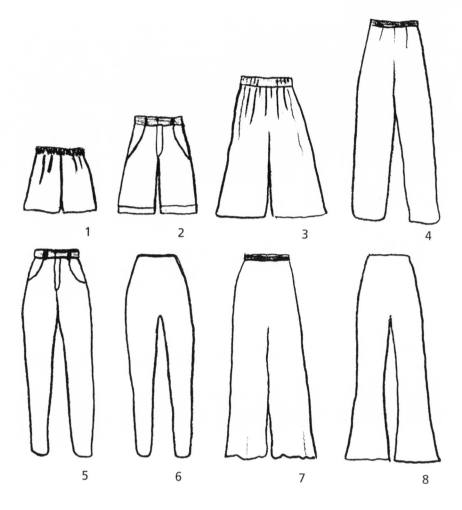

1   2   3   4

5   6   7   8

YOUR CLOTHING LOOK

You now have an understanding of what looks best for your figure. You have learned that the dictates of the fashion industry may not be right (every time) for you. Here's a checklist of clothing looks. Check off the items that are best for you. To look great, try not to deviate from the basic lines that work best for you.

	Yes	No	Possible
Garment Lines			
Horizontal	☐	☐	☐
Straight	☐	☐	☐
Curved	☐	☐	☐
Diagonal	☐	☐	☐
Vertical	☐	☐	☐
Garment Style			
Classic	☐	☐	☐
Avant-garde	☐	☐	☐
Romantic	☐	☐	☐
Country Casual	☐	☐	☐
Garment Details			
Blousy	☐	☐	☐
Clinging	☐	☐	☐
Ruffles	☐	☐	☐
Bows	☐	☐	☐
Pleats	☐	☐	☐
Large prints	☐	☐	☐
Small prints	☐	☐	☐
Heavily textured	☐	☐	☐
Smooth	☐	☐	☐
Pockets	☐	☐	☐

Garment Material

Wool	☐	☐	☐
Cotton	☐	☐	☐
Silk	☐	☐	☐
Linen	☐	☐	☐
Rayon	☐	☐	☐
Blends	☐	☐	☐
Velvet	☐	☐	☐
Lace	☐	☐	☐
Leather	☐	☐	☐
Faux fur	☐	☐	☐

Remember, you can look contemporary or modern without being a slave to the dictates of designers.

Choose the hem lengths that flatter your stature and legs. Have different lengths for different styles. Some skirts look better if they are long, some better if they are shorter. I have several hem lengths in my closet. And I wear them all. Anytime.

That's fun.

And fashionable.

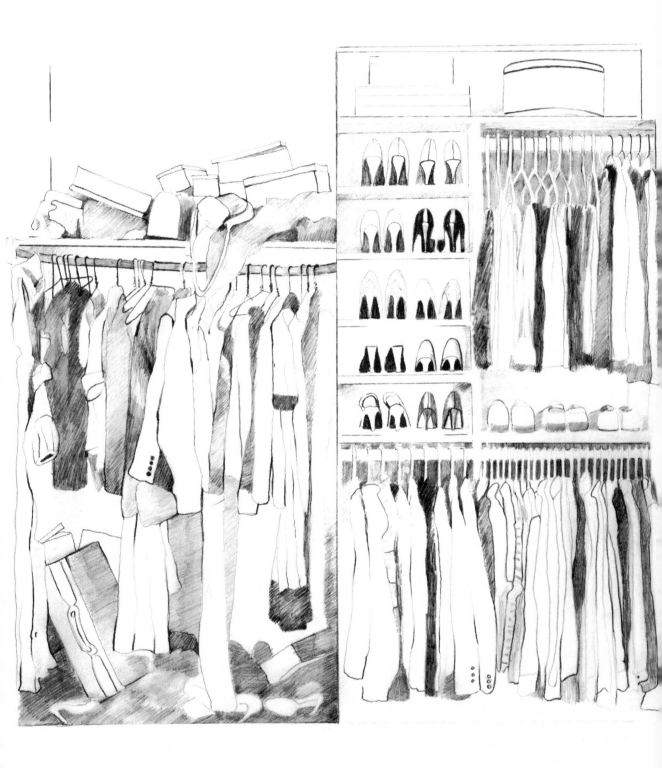

CHAPTER TEN

Clutter's Last Stand

How to Slim Down Your Wardrobe

"But dahling, *my closet is never cluttered."*

—Zsa Zsa Gabor

Listen to this: *You only wear 20 percent of what's in your closet. So tell me: What are you doing with the other 80 percent?* You should *wear* (and love) everything that's in your closet.

A designer once told me that a woman's wardrobe need only be thirty-six inches in width. (I can imagine what Zsa Zsa Gabor's reaction would be to that! Her walk-in closet has enough room to open a dry cleaner's.) The problem is weeding out. What do you throw away? What do you keep? It's a puzzlement. Now, if you went to a friend's house and looked in her closet, it wouldn't be any problem. You'd say:

"That color is ghastly on you."

"What have you been saving that for, a cruise on the *Titanic?*"

"Ugh. That's got to go. Even the colors next to it don't like it."

"Why are you saving that size 8 dress?"

Then you get the answer: *"I love that dress.* I'll get back into it when I lose fifteen pounds." Closets should not be *hope chests.* As full-figured actress Jane Russell once said: "Saying you're not going shopping until you've lost thirty pounds is like saying you won't drive until you have a Rolls-Royce."

It is difficult to be objective about your own wardrobe. After all, how could you possibly throw away the dress you had on the day you shook hands with the governor? Surely you can't be expected to dump your honeymoon outfit in the garbage. Yes you can! Closets should not be museums. They should be full of the present and future, not the past.

Do you have "skeletons" in your closet? That's called *closet guilt.* It's all those mistakes, the impulse buys and special items you found reduced 50 percent at the department store. When you got them home, they didn't go with anything you had. Like that big coat (the one that makes you look like a water buffalo), or that green flowered jacket (that looks like it needs watering).

Your closet should not be a museum or a hope chest.

 Magic Trick

We cart into our homes four times more stuff than we get rid of. The golden rule: Every time you add something to your wardrobe, get rid of something old or rarely worn. Cluttered, crammed closets waste precious time while you're searching for the right outfit. They make you feel guilty every time you open them.

Cleaning a closet is akin to quitting a job or ending a relationship that no longer works. You need to tear down that "old building" before you can build a new one. Closets are like gardens that need to be weeded, trimmed, and pruned. Do yourself a favor and clean yours out. You'll feel like you've taken a giant step toward a new you.

Once your closet is uncluttered and you have the right

things to wear for work and play, you'll be surprised how quickly you can get ready for any activity. No more trying on everything in your closet to see if it's right for the occasion or if you like it. You'll like it because you like everything in your closet.

HOW TO ORGANIZE YOUR CLOSET

Ten Things to Throw Out—Now!

- All those mistakes. Anything you thought you liked, wore once, and couldn't return. These are perfect for the consignment store.
- Things you haven't worn for a year.
- Basics that are seven to ten years old, like that blazer with the narrow lapels and the middle-of-the-rear length.
- All the clothes that no longer fit, the ones you are saving for the day you lose ten pounds. Every day you feel like a failure because you haven't shed the weight.
- Clothes with holes or tears you can't repair and stains that won't come out.
- The coat you've had for years and never wear (but was so expensive you're too guilty to get rid of).
- Lingerie that's died, like nylons with runs, bras that make you saggy, or panties that won't stay up without the help of safety pins.
- Shoes with gouged, rundown heels and scuffed toes, ratty belts and shabby scarves, jewelry you never wear.
- Old handbags that look worn and out of style.
- (This one's my favorite.) All the tacky clothes that make you look and feel like a slob, but which you are saving for the next time you paint the bathroom. One shabby outfit for summer and one for winter are all the grubby clothes you need to keep.

Now take all the clothes you haven't worn in a year (but can't bear to part with) and pack them into a box. Store the box in the attic or garage. In six months you won't remember what's in the box. Then give them to your favorite charity, or sell them at a garage sale. If the clothes look no older than two years and are in excellent condition, consider a consignment store.

Next, take all the items that need mending and get busy.

Check all the garments you've decided to keep and see if they're clean. It's amazing how many clothes "grow" stains right in the closet.

Now you're ready to put things back in the closet, sorted into these groups:

Dresses

Skirts

Pants

Blouses

Jackets

Separate the separates. Separate the suits, hanging all skirts together and all the jackets together. This will help you see new combinations.

Hang each group of blouses, pants, or dresses by color: black, gray, white, pink, red. This method will help you color coordinate with other items in the closet and do it quickly. No wire hangers. Use only plastic, padded, or wood.

Crocheted belt loops are meant to be used in the store to keep the outfit's belt on. They are tacky. Cut them off!

Complete the chart on the following pages with what you have left in each garment category:

WARDROBE INVENTORY CHART

Summer Items

Item	Shoes	Purses	Belts	Accessories

Dresses

1. _____
2. _____
3. _____
4. _____
5. _____

Skirts

1. _____
2. _____
3. _____
4. _____
5. _____

Pants

1. _____
2. _____
3. _____
4. _____
5. _____

Blouses

1. _____

2. _____

3. _____

4. _____

5. _____

Sweaters

1. _____

2. _____

3. _____

4. _____

5. _____

Jackets

1. _____

2. _____

3. _____

4. _____

5. _____

Coats

1. _____

2. _____

3. _____

4. _____

5. _____

Winter Items

Item	*Shoes*	*Purses*	*Belts*	*Accessories*

Dresses

1. _____
2. _____
3. _____
4. _____
5. _____

Skirts

1. _____
2. _____
3. _____
4. _____
5. _____

Pants

1. _____
2. _____
3. _____
4. _____
5. _____

Blouses

1. _____
2. _____
3. _____
4. _____
5. _____

Sweaters

1. _____
2. _____
3. _____
4. _____
5. _____

Jackets

1. _____
2. _____
3. _____
4. _____
5. _____

Coats

1. _____
2. _____
3. _____
4. _____
5. _____

Now list all the times you "didn't have a thing to wear" or felt overdressed or underdressed. Make a list of what you'd need for those activities and for other events that recur in your life. You only need one outfit for each different occasion. You don't go to the grocery store without a list, so don't go shopping without one. On a limited budget you will have to put a priority on what you want to buy first. To establish that priority remember your personal clothing lifestyle.

Professional The bulk of your clothing allowance should go into career clothes of the best quality you can afford. They should look like your boss's—you may be the boss someday.

Social If you are primarily a social person, then your closet should contain upscale casual clothes, suits, and dresses for luncheons, and for the evening, cocktail and evening gowns.

Homemaker If you are mainly a homebody or mom with children, then your closet should contain mostly casual clothes that make you look good but are practical as well. You want to feel that you look great all day long, too. (After all, being a homemaker is a job; the work just requires different clothes than a businesswoman wears.) You may need only one or two dressy outfits.

Spend the most dollars on what you spend the most hours doing. (Sleep doesn't count.)

THE BASIC WARDROBE

To achieve a basic, workable wardrobe will take time if you're counting the dollars, but you can afford what you want with careful planning. You cannot afford clothes you never wear, that are of poor quality, or that you don't love. Your basic pieces will be in the neutral tones of your color season and should be in solid colors, not prints. This way each item can be built upon and interchanged.

Jacket (1) This is the first building block in your wardrobe. The jacket must be classic, not faddish, and must be the best quality your budget will stand.

Skirts (2) One of the skirts may match the jacket or be in another neutral color. Both skirts need to be simple in style. One skirt should dress up (black knit, for instance).

Pants (2) May either match or contrast. Straight leg, not flared or tight. One pair can be in a casual jean style.

Dress (1) Basic, simple style that can be dressed up for evening or down for day. Plain, neutral color.

Blouses (3) You'll need three different styles: a casual shirt style (may be in print), a tailored basic to go with everything, and a dressy style that you can wear in the evening.

Sweaters (2) Try a cowl, turtleneck, or pullover that will go with pants and skirts. Also good is a cardigan (zipper or button) that you can use over your clothes for casual wear or cool weather.

Coat (1) Must be wearable for day as well as evening. A belted trench coat in a dressier fabric will take you almost anywhere.

Once you have completed this basic "survival" wardrobe, begin to add a casual jacket, casual skirt, more blouses (patterned or plain), T-shirts, and different sweaters. Then, by adding current accessories, you will have a timeless wardrobe that will require a little updating only twice a year—spring and fall.

When choosing clothes beyond your basic wardrobe, consider having only a few dresses and very few prints. You buy dresses because they are easy, especially print ones. You don't have to accessorize. That can also be extremely boring and limiting when all you can do is wear the dress over and over the same way. You can't change its look. Prints are also memorable to all your friends, and you will tire of them sooner. Plain classy colors (like a Mercedes) will take you farther and make you elegant.

THE SHOPPING SPREE

American women, as a rule, buy too many clothes of lesser quality. Take a tip from those chic French ladies. Even women on a small budget in France save their money to buy one great suit and always a fine handbag—and wear them to death. People who know quality will notice. It's far better to buy one quality outfit than two cheaper ones.

Who cares how many times you're seen in the same outfit, if you always look like you have a million in the bank? For that instant first impression there is nothing more important than your clothes. No one sees your house; few see your car. What they see are your clothes and jewelry.

Don't buy anything on sale you wouldn't pay full price for.

Go to the expensive stores. I didn't say *buy* at those stores. Just look. Use them as guides to what is fashionable and what is top quality. Then buy similar items in your price range at other stores, or wait for a sale.

At our Nordstrom department store I saw a pair of Ellen Tracy silk pants I truly wanted, but they were pricy. I asked the clerk to call me when they went on sale, then kept my fingers crossed, hoping that by that time they'd have a pair left in my size. She called. They did! I saved 50 percent.

A budget shopper gets many of her clothes at sales and discount stores. Prowl the consignment shops. You can find designer clothes at bargain basement prices.

If you need a good coat, you may have to wait until January to find one on sale. Don't freeze, plan ahead. Anticipate your needs a season earlier.

Sales can be a good deal, but *only* if the item is what you need and love. If not, and you find something that you know is perfect for you, pay the full price. It's like an investment: you'll get your money's worth because you'll wear it often and look and feel like a million.

A couple of seasons ago I found a gray wool pinstripe suit (jacket, pants, and skirt) that fit perfectly. I loved it, but it cost more than I had ever paid for a suit. It was the beginning of the season, so there was no chance it would be marked down. I gulped—and bought the skirt and jacket. A week later I gulped again—and bought the pants.

It was one of the best investments I ever made. I knew I looked classy in the outfit.

What you pay for a garment should be determined by how many times you'll wear it. I wore that suit two or three times a week. I took it on trips. I dressed it up for evening. I wore it for a day suit. *I still wear it.* By now the price per wearing is low—really low.

About eight years ago I bought a black St. John skirt—again a bit pricy. The knit is such good quality that it never sags or bags, even if I travel in it for hours, as I've done giving lectures and seminars. I've worn it with dressy tops for cocktails and with jackets for luncheons. I've worn it at least 200 times. You see, it was not really expensive, after all.

According to Ann Landers' "Gem of the Day," there are four reasons a woman buys an item of apparel:

It makes her look thin.
It was on sale.
Nobody else has one.
Everybody else has one.

To ensure that *you* buy right, check the following list:

- Go shopping by yourself. Friends are fun, but not always the best source of advice. *You* must decide what you like.
- Always go shopping when you are *not* tired.
- Don't go shopping in tennis shoes. They may be comfortable, but they won't get you good service.
- Carry shoes that will complement what you are looking for.
- Never be an impulse buyer, unless you know something is absolutely right for you.
- Don't shop at the last minute for an important

occasion. You'll end up paying more and liking what you buy less.
- Stick to your *basic wardrobe* list and try to fill the empty spaces in your closet. Go for the quality classic outfits that will upgrade your wardrobe. These are the pieces that will last for years. Buy natural fabrics or blends that look natural: wool, silk, cotton.

Magic Trick

Make sure the garment you buy fits *today,* not five pounds from today. No pulled pockets, pleats or buttons, please. The outfit should flow smoothly from your shoulders—tight enough to show you're a woman, loose enough to show you're a lady.

Here is a checklist to use when you shop:
- **Color** Don't look at colors that don't flatter.
- **Fabric** If it's not a fabric that flatters (too bulky, like linen, or too clingy like latex) then don't try it on.
- **Line/Design** If it won't enhance your body shape by its own shape, there is no need to try it on.
- **Cost** Buy the best you can afford, or even a little better than you can afford. Keep in mind how often you would wear it. If it's really basic—one of the building blocks of your wardrobe—be sure it's of excellent quality. Cost per wearing will be small: if you wear a $300 suit once a week for four years, that's $1.50 per wearing.
- **Coordination** Do you have other things to wear with the item? If not, you don't need it.
- **Cleaning instructions** Washable is affordable. Dry cleaning can add 100 percent to the cost. If it's off-white wool that needs cleaning almost every time you wear it, think again about buying. Some items that say "Dry Clean Only" can

be washed by hand, such as silks and linens. Many manufacturers label their garments with this note so they don't have to be responsible if you don't wash them properly.

Magic Trick

If shopping isn't your thing and you're never sure what to buy, try a "personal shopper." Many department stores offer these services, which are free and without obligation. The personal shopper will schedule an appointment so she can meet with you to determine your needs and budget. The shopper will gather items for you, put you in a large dressing room, and help you choose what is right for your color and shape. If nothing is to your liking, the shopper will watch for things you might be interested in, then call you. Since there is no obligation or fee for this service, there is no better way to avoid making costly mistakes than getting professional help.

TRAVELING WITH EASE

Once you have revitalized your closet, you'll be surprised how simple and quick it is to pack for that special weekend. Everything is coordinated. Everything will fit into one bag.

Times have changed since the following tips on "How to Go Abroad" were published in a magazine by the "Miss Manners" of the 1880s.

For your traveling dress: wear wool and quiet colors or you will look "vulgar."

Cover your hat with brown paper to keep your ostrich plumes dry.

The Miss Manners of today would simply say: "Unclutter today!"

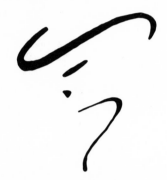

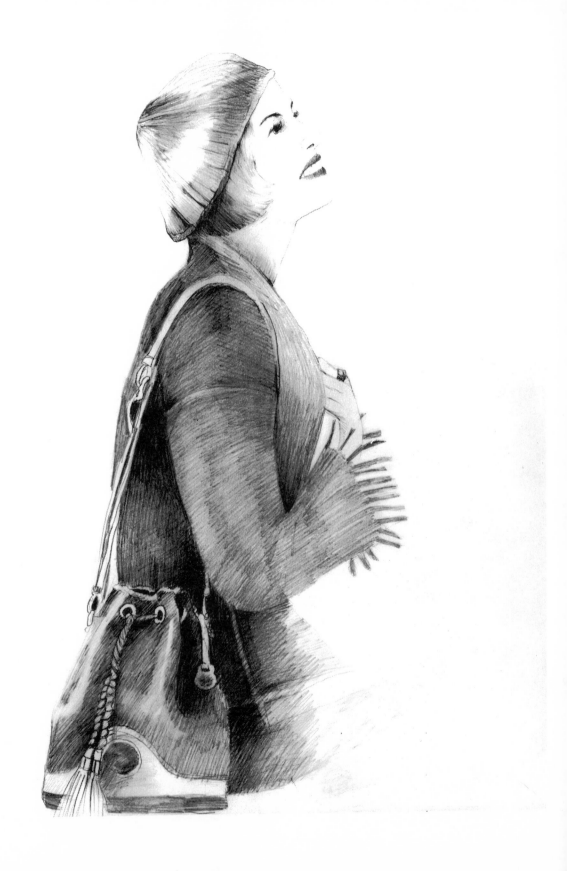

CHAPTER ELEVEN

Baubles, Bangles, and Beads

Choosing the Right Accessories

"Elegance is the art of not astonishing."

—Jean Cocteau

Finally. You're beginning to feel that you can fool the world with clothes that flatter your figure—but you're not quite through yet. It's time to take a look at accessories.

You're in charge of what catches someone's eye when they look at you. The eye is naturally drawn first to metal (jewelry or belts). Next it sees lace. So if you'd rather people didn't notice your hips, don't wear a large metal buckle (unless you have a jacket on). Wear your metal around your neck and on your ears. Tuck that lace hanky in your breast pocket. Wear a lace teddy or blouse under your suit jacket. Put a lamé scarf around your neck.

Accessories are important. They can:
- Make simple clothes stand out in a different way each time they are worn
- Make a cheap outfit look richer
- Create excitement and individuality in your wardrobe
- Update an old outfit

If your outfit is chic, elegant, or quiet, don't jar the mood by accessorizing with too bright a scarf or jewelry. Keep the mood. You can use startling accessories and bright colors with fun clothes.

Shoes, stockings, purses, jewelry, scarves, belts, and hats add style and class to your first impression image.

Magic Trick

The right color stocking can appear to change your leg size. The style of a shoe can make your legs look longer and thinner, or shorter and wider. Let accessories be part of your disguise.

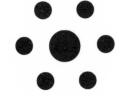

Figure 1

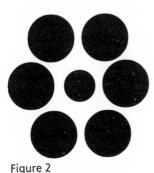

Figure 2

Proportion

Which center dot is larger? You're right. They're both the same. What does that tell you? If you're a large person (figure 1) you'd better get over there and hang out with the extra large people (figure 2). As the old joke goes, "If you want to look thinner, just hang out with fat people."

It's all about proportion. I once had a student who was a large-boned woman. She always wore tiny earrings. I asked her why. She replied, "Because I have a large face, and large earrings would make my face look larger." Wrong. Her face would look *smaller* if she wore large jewelry, as illustrated in Figure 2. Upon my advice she started using larger jewelry, and it worked.

The opposite is true of the petite person who looks smaller because she is overwhelmed by her accessories. Be sure your accessories are in proportion to your size. If your purse is so large you look like you need a bellhop to carry it, then you should scale down.

ACCESSORIES

Handbags

Grandma called them pocketbooks. Mom called them purses. We call them handbags.

The old rule for a handbag—the earlier the hour the larger the bag; the later the hour, the smaller the bag—still holds true. You don't want to plop a luggage-size tote bag on the dinner table of an elegant restaurant.

The size of the bag is important in looking great. Keep it in proportion to your stature. If you are short or petite, don't let your body be overpowered by your bag. If you are Junoesque, then go big.

We are all different heights, yet we buy a shoulder bag and wear it, no matter the length. If you can curl your fingers under the bottom of the bag when shouldering it, the length is right. If it's knocking on your knees or hanging below your hemline, it's too long. Adjust the buckle if it has one. Tie a knot in the strap if it doesn't. Or better yet, take it to a shoe repair shop for adjustment.

If your hips are large, don't dangle a shoulder bag there. It will add bulk. Carry it just above the hip line.

Handbags are like closets: the larger they are, the more we stuff inside them.

Handbags are like closets: the larger they are, the more we stuff inside them. And look at all the extra weight we have to carry around, adding a lopsided look to those shoulders. Get rid of the nonessentials. Carry only what you need: makeup, billfold, glasses, and keys. If you can't bear to leave things at home, put all those extra items in a tote and leave it in the car. Your handbag should be large enough to hold essentials without looking bulgy.

Ever wonder what Queen Elizabeth II carries in that little bag she always has on her person? No one really knows, but my guess is makeup and glasses. I doubt she carries money, an ID card, or the keys to Buckingham Palace.

Your handbag can match your shoes or blend with them but it should never be darker than the shoes. Your bag should also blend with the outfit you're wearing. Be careful with textured bags;

they simply don't go with very many things. The plainer, the more practical. If you buy a bag in your basic seasonal colors, it will coordinate with most of your wardrobe.

Buy bags with little (or preferably no) silver or gold ornamentation. The extra metal shows wear faster and can look too busy.

Invest in one good daytime bag that will go with the majority of your wardrobe. People recognize a quality bag. It will not only look great, it will make you feel good for years.

When you do change bags for an outing, have the little things in small bags so it will be simple to transfer everything: makeup and comb together; tissue in a packet; pen in a billfold.

Never carry a briefcase and a handbag at the same time.

Belts

Belts add a finishing touch. They can also make a fashion statement and give the illusion of sleekness.

You don't have to have a tiny waist to wear a belt.

If you are thick-waisted, don't wear a stark, contrasting color; it attracts attention to the middle of your body. For a slimming effect, wear a color that blends with your outfit, and choose a belt that isn't too wide.

Chain belts are good for wearing loosely around larger waists. You can angle a belt from the center waist to the hip. Angles of any kind are slimming, so try slipping the buckle off center.

Unless you're slim, don't cinch a belt tightly around your waist; wear it loosely or just below the waist. (I can't recall how many times I've seen women use a wide belt as a girdle, only to have a roll of fat squeeze out like putty.)

Are you long waisted, short waisted or average? This determines the width of belt you can wear. The longer waisted, the wider the belt; the shorter waisted, the narrower the belt.

To make yourself appear longer waisted, match the belt to your blouse. To appear shorter waisted, match the belt to your skirt.

Elastic waistbands need to be covered with a top worn outside, blousoned over the waistband, or with a belt.

Why not use a scarf or sash as a belt? Loop a bangle bracelet though a scarf to make a buckle. Scarves can also be tied loosely just below the waist.

Hats

Wearing a hat creates an excellent first impression. The observer believes you have self-confidence. People will not look and say, "Who does she think she is?" They'll think, "I wish I could do that. She looks wonderful."

Don't just envy hats on someone else. Wear one. I guarantee you'll receive compliments.

Hats are fun.

In Santa Barbara, the Polo & Racquet Club holds an annual afternoon event called "The Great Gatsby." Celebrities and just plain folk flock to the party in elegant cars and costumes. The women are ready for the Gatsby gala on the lawn in their large feminine hats.

Hats are practical.

They help keep the sun off your face. Buy a simple wide-brimmed hat and create your own style. Tie a brilliant scarf around the brim, add flowers, feathers, or a wisp of lace. You'll look like Princess Di at the Ascot races.

Try a gambler or western hat to wear with jeans and casual clothes. Use a visor or a baseball cap—a fashion statement and a sun shade at the same time.

There are hat styles for everyone, but not every style is right for all people. If you have a full figure, you should wear a hat in proportion to your size. If you wear a tiny pillbox hat, you'll look like you have a huge aspirin on your head.

The brim of a hat should not be wider than your shoulders. The crown should be as wide as the widest part of your face. Look at the back view as well as the front. That's what others see.

Please, no long hair dangling from a dressy hat. On her husband's 1992 inaugural day on the steps of the capitol, Hillary Clinton wore a ponytail hanging out of her hat. Tacky, tacky. Wear

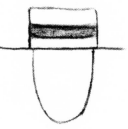

Sailor

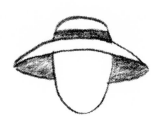

Cloche

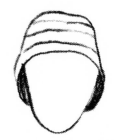

Cartwheel

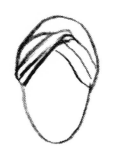

Turban

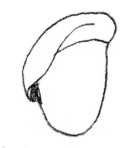

Beret

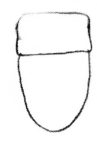

Pillbox

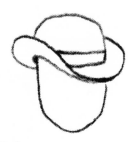

Derby

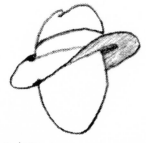

Fedora

your long hair up. Save the long hair and ponytails for cowboy hats, berets, and caps. Likewise, dangling earrings don't usually look good with hats, either.

Faces are not symmetrical, so most hats shouldn't sit squarely on the head. Leave that to Smokey the Bear. To look elegant or chic (instead of silly), wear large dress hats and cowboy hats low on your forehead, so you can just see out. You don't want to look like a Holly Hobby little girl with your hat tipped back on your head.

To avoid chasing the hat if the wind picks up, try a hat pin. Pierce the hat with the pin, twist it around a hunk of hair, then push the pin back out. If there's an elastic strap, it goes under your hair, not your chin.

Heads are not all the same size. Neither are hats. Be sure to get one large enough to rest comfortably on your forehead.

Good hats are stored in boxes, not perched on a hat rack where they get dusty and lose shape.

Never chew gum in a veiled hat!

Shoes

Shoes are one of the most important accessories you can wear. No matter how perfect your outfit, hair, and makeup, if you wear the wrong shoes, you will have ruined your entire look. It's better to keep your old outfit and update your shoes than to buy a new dress and wear improper, outdated, or shabby footwear.

Shoes should never be lighter in color than your hemline. One exception is when you neutralize your whole leg by wearing taupe or nude stockings and a taupe or camel shoe. Then your shoe can be lighter than your hemline because it's an extension of your leg. When a model's tote bag doesn't have exactly the right color of shoe to go with red or royal blue, she'll use this neutralizing trick.

Magic Trick

Never wear white pumps with anything but white unless you want to look like Minnie Mouse. Tennis shoes don't count. Instead of white shoes, try metallic, gold, silver, pewter, or black patent with white. Off-white, winter white, or cream shoes can be worn with clothes that have these colors in the print. You might wear pastel shoes. If you're trying to decide whether to wear a light or dark shoe with an outfit, go dark.

You'll look taller (and your legs slimmer) if you blend your shoe and hose color into your skirt color.

If you want to wear a brightly colored shoe such as red, pink, or yellow, be sure you don't have more than one other accessory item in the same bright color. (Earrings don't count.) You can wear a scarf or belt or purse of the same bright color as the shoes, but never all three.

If your legs are plump, pumps with a low vamp will slim them. Any strap across the foot or at the ankle widens the leg. Heels add length to the leg and give an illusion of slimness. But don't go so high you look like you're wearing stilts. Wedgies are good for casual wear instead of totally flat shoes to add slimness and height.

Boots are a great fashion statement and totally camouflage a full leg or a skinny one. One rule: Never, *never* allow space between the top of the boot and your skirt or pants, unless it's a miniskirt and boots. If you buy only one pair of boots, be sure they are high enough to come under all of your skirts. Also, they should be in a neutral color, to coordinate with a variety of outfits. Boots come in flat and high heels, sporty to dressy, and can be extremely practical and comfortable. They're wonderful with long skirts. You can be wearing boots and looking smart when everyone else is in tennis shoes. Collect them whenever your budget allows.

You can add years to your age by wearing matronly shoes. There are lots of shoe styles that are both comfortable and good looking. Don't settle for less.

Stockings

Light hose make your legs look larger; dark hose make your legs look thinner. Stockings are never darker than your shoe.

If you have full legs, avoid textured hose, regardless what fashion or fads decree. The exception is if the texture is in a slimming vertical line. If your legs are slim, play with texture to achieve the right effect. Textured hose often draw attention to the area you are trying to disguise. Beware of lace-patterned hose that make you look like you have leprosy. No white hose unless you are a nurse. The same goes for hose the color of heavy cream.

A nude stocking should match your arms in color. No suntanned legs and white arms, please. For a leg-slimming look, blend your hose color with your skirt and shoes.

Don't wear reinforced toes showing in open-toe shoes. Wear knee-high hose with a dress only if you're going to a Halloween party as a Girl Scout.

If you wear pantyhose with slacks and jeans, you will eliminate panty line. Bulges around panties add pounds—even on skinny women. Try thong panties instead.

Hose will fit better if you buy the kind that don't have a foot shape woven in. The hose will assume the shape of your foot and leg. If your stockings bag, buy a better brand with more latex.

Stockings should be *de rigueur* for dress pumps. Save bare toes for sandals or mules.

Jewelry

Do you like classic jewelry, real gold, and pearls? Or do you prefer to show your creativity with costume jewelry? I like both. Of course, on a limited budget, who can afford a pound of gold hanging around one's neck? A strand of cultured pearls is a lovely accessory, but expensive. If you like classic jewelry, save your pennies for special pieces. Meanwhile, you can use "genuine simulated" jewelry.

Costume jewelry can be fun!

You can spark up an outfit with some reasonably priced contemporary baubles. Color and style can make up for the expensive price tag. Be a bargain hunter. Look for sales. Check out consignment stores and antique clothing stores for retro jewelry.

I'm a swap-meet and garage-sale junkie. I hover over tables of costume jewelry. I have collected a drawerful of earrings, another of bracelets and necklaces. It's okay to mix the authentic and not-so-authentic.

Now here's a few hints on wearing jewelry.

If you are a large or big-boned woman, don't wear dainty jewelry. Use large pieces to complement your size. Wear several bangles instead of just one, large rings on large fingers.

When shopping, remember your color season's metals: silver, white gold, platinum, or rose gold for Summers and Winters; gold and copper for Springs and Autumns. Do mix metals. That gold necklace that is not in your color tone can be blended with a silver one that is. Wear gold and silver bangles at the same time. Two-toned watches are a great way to tie two jewelry colors together.

Do mix metals. That gold necklace that is not in your color tone can be blended with a silver one that is.

Consider your face shape when you buy large earrings or drop earrings. Flatter your face with jewelry that doesn't repeat your face shape.

If your face is round, don't accentuate it with round button earrings. Choose another shape.

If your face is long, don't make it longer with drop earrings.

If your face is oval, do anything you want.

The texture and weight of jewelry should be compatible with the texture of the fabric you're wearing. The style should also be compatible. If you have a romantic dress, you won't put tailored Chanel jewelry with it. Use something delicate. If you're wearing a classic outfit, you can use classic or dramatic jewelry.

A special piece of jewelry or an elaborate belt can be the *focal point* of your whole outfit. In that case, let it stand alone. Only add simple things that don't stand in the way of the distinctive piece. Jewelry can also be the *finishing* touch to an outfit, and then you can use several pieces.

Please, no matching earring, bracelet, and necklace sets. You'll look like you came from a cookie cutter. Only wear two matching pieces, or no matching pieces.

Don't always feel, as many of my students do, that you must wear a necklace. Many times, earrings are all you need. There is something pretty about a bare neck.

 Magic Trick

You can look taller and thinner and lengthen a short neck by wearing long necklaces. Chokers and short necklaces work with long necks and thin women.

Glasses

What do people see first on your face? Glasses. If you wear them, this is not the place to budget. Buy the best and most attractive you can afford. Go to a knowledgeable licensed optician who understands not only the technical aspects, but also style.

Glasses should never duplicate the face shape. They should be as wide as the widest part of your face and follow the contour of your eyebrows, bisecting the brow in half. The only exception is the vintage 1920 and '30s style of small round glasses. Eyebrows shouldn't show completely through the lens.

A high or rounded bridge on the glasses is good for a small nose; a lower straight bridge for a long nose.

If your face is long, get a bow (the ear piece) that's placed mid-line into the frame front, not at the top where the eyebrow ends. This shortens the face.

Buy glasses in the metal that flatters your skin.

Cosmetic tints are passe in clear lenses. Be sure your sunglasses are tinted in a color that complements your skin tone. Do have UVA and UVB protective coating on your sunglasses to protect your eyes from harmful rays that can lead to cataracts.

Magic Trick
Try a no-glare coating on your clear lens. That way people can see right into your beautifully made up eyes. It's worth the extra dollars, and you'll love it.

Underwear

If you can only have one color bra or panties what should it be? That's right, nude, the color closest to your skin tone. It won't show under white, as white underwear will.

Are you still wearing a slip with all your dresses? Why? Because your mother told you to? Most of the time you don't need one. The less underneath, the less that will show: no more slips peeking though slits in skirts, or slips showing a line shorter than the skirt hem.

If you see a total leg outline through the dress, you might need a slip. Perhaps opaque stockings or tights would work better. Some new skirts are meant to show legs. With knit skirts that cling, a slip will soften the line. Otherwise, save your money and don't wear slips.

Tuck your shirt tails into your panty hose. You'll get a smoother line, and the tail won't show through the skirt.

If bra straps show on a low neckline, put a safety pin in the shoulder of the blouse, run the strap through the loop of the pin without attaching it, and close the safety pin.

Scarves

Do you feel you were born without a scarf-tying gene? You weren't. You're only limited by a lack of imagination, and you're left with a drawer full of scarves you never wear. I constantly hear women say, "I can't tie scarves. They look terrible on me." You *can* tie scarves and they *won't* look terrible. It only takes a little help to get started.

The longer I work with scarves, the more I know there are

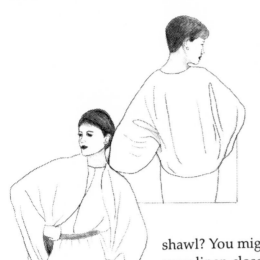

Butterfly Wrap

limitless ways to tie them. (They are also a great way to camouflage problem areas, because they divert the eye.)

One of the most successful fashion seminars I give on cruise ships is scarf-tying. Not only are the women enthralled by the creative ways a colorful piece of material can be used to liven up an outfit and "tie" it together, they are shocked by the simplicity of the craft.

Have you ever used one of your cloth napkins as a scarf? (Just be careful it doesn't have a gravy stain on it.) How about using a tablecloth as a shawl? You might be surprised at the wearable accessories hiding in your linen closet.

I was once desperate for an evening wrap and got the bright idea to wear a hand-crocheted antique bed coverlet as a shawl. It looked great, but by the end of the evening I felt like I had on a suit of armor. (If you've ever lifted crochet work you know how heavy it can be.) I wasn't wearing a doily, I was wearing a bedspread. I put it back on the bed and haven't worn it since.

Magic Trick

I always start a scarf-tying demonstration with this trick that is right out of a magician's hat. Instead of wearing a shawl like Granny Goose by draping it over each shoulder, take a crocheted tablecloth or large square (54") of fabric and fold it in half with the wrong side out. Tie the two ends together on each side. Open to the right side and slip your arms through the openings. It's called the "Butterfly Wrap" and it makes a clever day or evening accessory. Use it for those times when you've gone through the closet to find a jacket or coat and nothing matches, or everything's the wrong length. You don't want to go to a party looking tacky, nor do you want to freeze. Use the Butterfly Wrap to keep the chill off.

Scarves are great budget savers to update something old. During my scarf demonstrations I wear a basic black dress that I bought half-price several years ago. (Talk about pennies per wearing!) I demonstrate the many ways to tie scarves on that old dress to make it contemporary.

If you have a short neck, you can still wear scarves. Just don't use bulky fabrics, and tie the scarf lower.

Remove the labels manufacturers love to sew into scarves, and you're ready to begin. It's a simple and easy art to tie scarves. First learn the four basic folds.

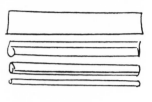

Oblong Fold

FOUR BASIC SCARF FOLDS

The Oblong Fold Take a long scarf, fold one side one-third up, then fold the opposite side to overlap, then fold once more.

The Triangle Fold Fold one corner of a square scarf to the opposite corner. Overlap the hem by two inches.

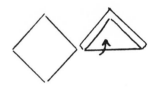

Triangle Fold

The Square into a Long Fold Fold a corner of a square scarf up a few inches beyond the corner of the material. Fold the top corner down, then keep folding to desired width. Long necks need a wider scarf, short necks a narrower one.

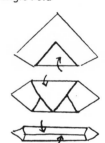

Accordion Pleat Fold Lay out the scarf on a table and fold it like an accordion or a Japanese fan.

Square into Long Fold

Accordion Pleat Fold

ONE BASIC KNOT

Square Knot Put a folded scarf around your neck, with one side hanging over the other. Tie the top end over the bottom. Create a loop, then bring the top end through loop. Pull through the opening.

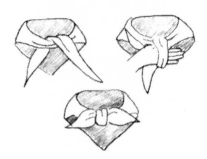

CLASSIC NECK SCARVES (LARGE SQUARES)

Dog Collar Use an oblong fold. Put around neck with ends in the back. Cross ends to the front. Tie a square knot.

Turtle Fold a square scarf into a triangle. Put over mouth, wrap around head, and tie in the front. Cuff over scarf to hide knot. Pull down to neck.

Paper Fan Accordion pleat a square scarf. Either tie and fan out around the neck, or tie to a pony tail.

Bib Knot Spread out a square scarf wrong side up and knot the center. Turn right side out and it will magically look like a butterfly. Tie corners around the neck.

Scouting Tie Fold a square scarf into a triangle. Tie with a square knot. Put the knot in the front, back, or on the side.

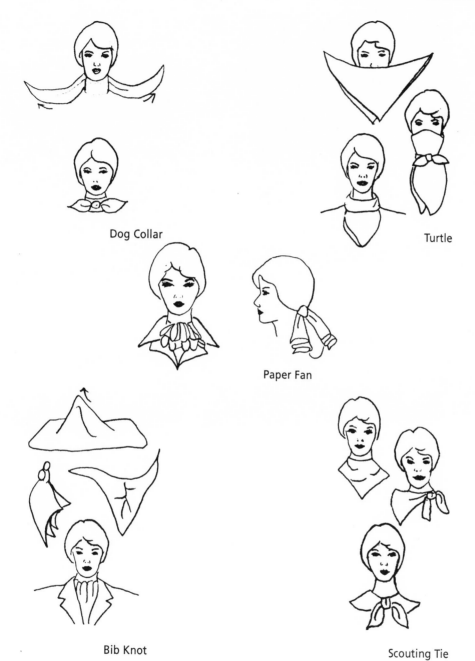

Dog Collar

Turtle

Paper Fan

Bib Knot

Scouting Tie

CLASSIC NECK SCARVES (OBLONG)

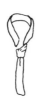 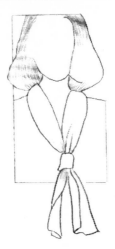

Slip Knot Place an oblong or bias scarf around the neck with one end longer than the other. Tie a simple knot in the longer end. Place the other end into and through the knot and tighten slightly. This tie makes you look taller and thinner.

Oblong Wrap Place the center of an oblong or bias scarf in the front. Cross the ends behind the neck and back to the front, leaving the ends loose.

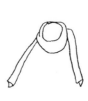 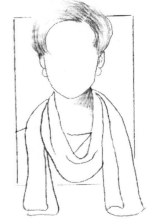

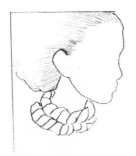

Oblong Knot Wrap an oblong scarf around the neck. Tie once. Twist ends separately. Cross ends over at neck. Wrap to back of neck and tie in a knot.

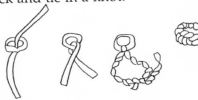

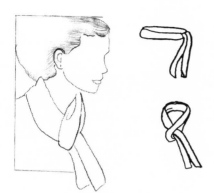

Hacking Knot Take an oblong scarf and fold it in half. Put around the neck and pull the ends through the loop. Pull up as tight as desired.

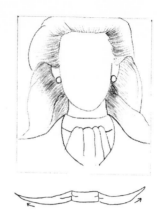

Ascot Use an oblong scarf and wrap it around the neck. Cross the ends and bring them to the front. Flip one end over the other.

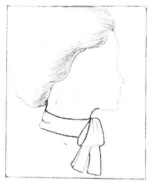 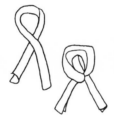

The Puff Take an oblong scarf and cross one end over the other, keeping one end longer. Then tie. Take a longer end and pull part way through, then puff out the material.

The Rosette Place an oblong scarf around the neck and make a secure double knot close to the neck. Twist both ends together until the scarf coils. Wrap the scarf around the knot and tuck both ends behind the rosette.

   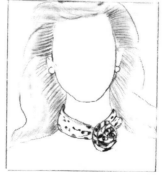

CLASSIC HEAD SCARVES

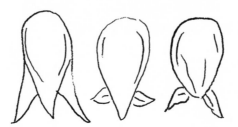

Turban #1 Fold a square scarf into a triangle. Knot in the back under the point, then tuck point under the knot.

Turban #2 Fold a large square scarf into a triangle, then cross the ends in back and bring them to the front and knot.

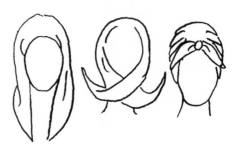

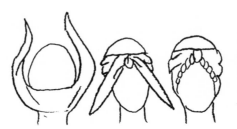

Turban #3 Use an oblong scarf. Place it around the back of the head, wrap and knot in front. Twist the ends and tuck under the side.

Head Wrap Fold a square scarf into a triangle and place on head. Cross the ends in front, bring them to the back and tie scarf over the point. For another look, simply secure the ends under the chin.

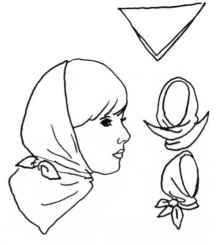

SHAWL DRESSING

Throw Fold the shawl into triangle and put around the shoulders, and toss one end over the other shoulder.

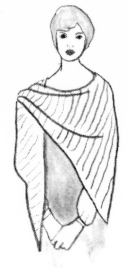

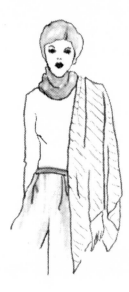

Drape Fold the shawl in a triangle and simply drape over one shoulder.

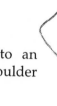

Knotted Fold the shawl into an oblong shape, put it over one shoulder diagonally and knot near the waist.

Magic Trick

Scarves will not stay in place like magic. Use straight-pins to hold them in place, not safety pins. You can also pin with a decorative piece of jewelry.

TWENTY HANDY ACCESSORY HINTS

1. Intertwine two contrasting colors of neck beads into one strand. Twist or braid two scarves together.
2. String a large wooden bead (purchased at a craft shop) on a scarf and tie around your neck. It's smart looking and guaranteed to get compliments.
3. Clip earrings on shoes.
4. Combine different chains in silver, gold, and crystal.
5. Combine different plastic, wood, and metal bracelets.
6. Use a scarf around a hat for a hat band, and pin with a pierced earring.
7. Wear two clip-on earrings together. Creates a dramatic look.
8. Turn the neck of your blouse under and tie a scarf for a new neckline.
9. Wear a blouse or sweater backward for a different neckline.
10. Hang a long contrasting scarf around your raincoat collar for color interest.
11. Pin flowers of leather or silk on blouses and dresses.
12. Turn up your blazer collar and pin a flower on the back of the lapel.
13. Use an old ring or pin to loop a scarf through.
14. Change the buttons on a sweater or blouse for a new look, or to make a bargain look classy.
15. If your shoulders are narrow or sloped, attach shoulder pads with Velcro in all tops, including blouses.
16. Shop in the boys' and men's departments for shirts, sweaters, and vests—for you. They are frequently cheaper.
17. Put a piece of lace around your neck and pin on your grandmother's cameo.
18. Wear lace with denim. Add a lace scarf to your favorite denim skirt and blouse. Try wearing a lace blouse with a leather skirt.
19. Put a long scarf through a bangle bracelet and pin the end. Use as a belt by putting the other end though the bangle and tying or pinning.
20. Buy a scarf clip and use it for even more scarf variations.

16-POINT SYSTEM TO AVOID OVERDRESSING

Most women I see in my seminars and classes are under-accessorized. If you don't have an artist's eye to judge yourself, then here's a point system that works. It's a guide, not the Bible.

Sixteen points is a good median. A total count from 14 to 17 is good. Less than 11 points and you're under-dressed. If you score 18 points or more, you're wearing too much. (Exception—avant-garde people can have a count in the mid-20s.)

Five points for each item if plaid, check, striped, or patterned:

___ Suit
___ Dress
___ Shirt

___ Coat
___ Scarf

Two points each item:

___ Two-tone watch
___ Earrings or bracelet
___ Handbag with metal trim
___ Rings with stones or detail

___ Two-tone shoes, contrasting
    detail or straps
___ Textured hose

One point for each item:

___ Buttons (in contrasting color; plain buttons: zero)
___ Plain ring, watch, earring
___ Basic shoes
___ Blending hose

___ Plain suit, skirt, sweater
    dress, pants, or handbag

Use your imagination when wearing accessories. Be artistic. Dare to dare! You'll feel proud when complimented on an outfit you accessorized so creatively. It's just one more trick to looking great instantly that you have pulled out of your magician's hat.

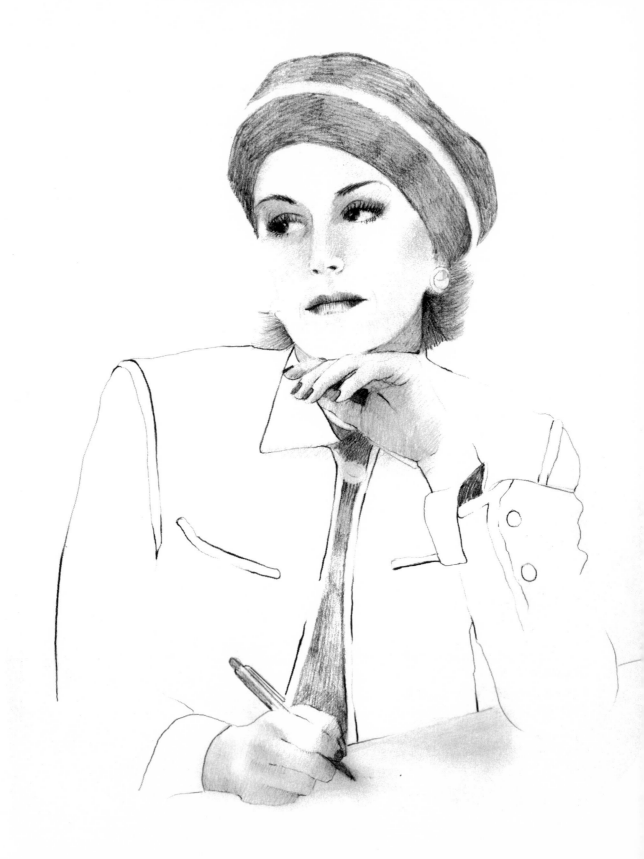

CHAPTER TWELVE

The Classic Woman:

Fabulous at Forty, Fantastic at Fifty, Sensational at Sixty

Looking Vibrant at Any Age

> *"I shall die very young. How young? I don't know, maybe seventy, maybe eighty, maybe ninety. But I shall be very young."*
>
> —Jeanne Moreau

Grandma shoes.

I always think of printed aprons and "grandma shoes" when classifying the stereotypical old woman. They're the kind of things my grandmother used to wear.

When I was twenty-one, I thought everyone over forty was *old*. Then I met a marvelous seventy-nine-year-old woman who was young at heart. "I'm too young to be old," she told me. She had painted her apartment purple and wore a low-cut purple blouse with pants and drove a tiny pink sports car when nobody even *owned* sports cars. She wasn't eccentric, she was simply vibrant—and wonderful.

I have always liked this quote from movie sex symbol Burt Reynolds: "Most women don't come into their own until thirty-five, and don't know who they are until they're forty-five. Women over thirty-five are tremendously interesting to me; over forty-five, fascinating; over fifty, irresistible.... For me a young woman is a pretty little pattern, an older woman, a kaleidoscope."

Fortunately for the women of this decade, the stigma of being classified "old" at forty or fifty or sixty (or even seventy) has passed into the dustbin of history, along with "grandma shoes."

Having passed the half-century mark, I like to think of myself as a "classic woman." (My modeling agency classifies me, with my silver hair, as a "classic" model.) That doesn't mean they have to give me a new paint job and stand me against a Rolls-Royce to make me look good. It means I'm a woman who will never stop experimenting with her own style and continuing to refine it.

You can be a

role model

at any age.

And we are *not* senior citizens, nor are we old. As the saying goes, we are *time honored,* or, if you prefer, *chronologically advantaged.*

Gustave Flaubert once said, "No sooner do we come into this world than bits of us start to fall off." That may be how you feel as you reach mid-life, but staying young has much less to do with the actual years in which we measure our lives than how we take care of ourselves and feel about ourselves. Age isn't chronological; age is a state of mind, an attitude. It has to do with the energy we project, whether we walk tall with good posture and carriage, speak vibrantly, have curiosity, and most importantly, have a sense of humor. I've known women who are old at thirty, and women young at sixty. A positive attitude will take off years. We may not be able to keep all of our parts from falling off, but we can get a new tune up every now and then.

In talking with thousands of women while teaching beauty classes and conducting seminars, I've discovered that too many are self-conscious about their ages. Even women in their early forties. The tell me they are too *old* to improve themselves, too old to go to school, too old to learn something new.

I say to them—Try it! Shoot for your dreams. As greeting card designer Flavia says, "Those who reach, touch the stars." Don't worry about the age of others. Let the younger women learn from your experience, while you learn from the energy of their youth. You can be a role model at any age. As Burt Reynolds said, "A woman gains a certain attractiveness with the confidence, success, and achievement that come with age."

Actresses like Jane Fonda and Joan Collins have tried to demystify getting older. The have blazed an enviable trail by looking young, healthy, and sexy into their forties, fifties, and sixties—and they'll look great into their seventies. As front-runners in the struggle for women to be acceptable and vibrant human beings at any age, they, and women like them, have made a significant contribution.

They have given maturing women new goals, new dreams, something to aim for and shout about. Our society is so youth-oriented that we need these public figures to make us aware that youth isn't all there is. Being young is an act of nature. Being old is a work of art.

Being young is an act of nature.

Being old is a work of art.

To be a vibrant woman of today, you must be healthy, have energy, and not worry about trying to mirror an unattainable image of youth, glamour, and perfection. The last thing a mature woman should do is try to hang on to an image from her youth. That pompadour hairdo that you loved and made you look so good in the 1940s is not for you now.

Forget your fifties pageboy, or the sixties ironed hair, or the seventies balloon bouffant. If you're still wearing that beehive hairdo teased to the maximum, you are out of sync with the times, and that spells A-G-I-N-G.

Aging by denial just doesn't work.

How many times have you looked at a woman from the back, someone with a mane of red hair and an attractive figure, and made an immediate mental judgment: that person is thirty, maybe thirty-five. Then she turns around. The makeup is a garish mask of heavy foundation, brilliant eyeliner, and red, red lipstick that highlights the wrinkles. And the hair is badly dyed. Underneath that clown's mask of makeup and plastic hair is a woman of sixty *trying to look young.* It just doesn't work.

Find your own style and stick with it. Style never goes out of fashion. Sure, you have to make subtle shifts that update your look, but the idea is to keep up with the times and not worry about birthdays.

Skin Care for the Classic Woman

"The older you get, the more it takes to look the way you want to," explains Trish McEvay, makeup artist from New York. "The challenge is for it to look effortless."

Classic women practically always have dry skin. Wrinkles show more when your skin is dry, so it's doubly important to moisturize. You may need a richer moisturizer for nighttime in addition to your regular one for day. Here are some helpful hints for skin care:

- Classic women must use sunscreen on any patch of skin that is subjected to the sun—face, arms, legs, hands.
- Check out the age reducing creams: Retin A and AHAs described in the makeup chapter.
- Try Cetaphil as a facial cleanser because it is non-drying.

Makeup Tips for the Classic Woman

"As the signs of aging increase, the natural look that may have served you so well in your thirties won't work in your forties," says Barbara Salomone, president of Bioelements, a makeup and skincare company. But, she warns, don't fall into the trap of using heavy foundation to hide things. It can settle into lines and wrinkles, making them show more. A damp sponge can give a lighter touch to foundation application.

If your skin is very dry, you may need an oil-based foundation instead of water-based to keep that moist look. You want light to medium coverage, not heavy.

Use your green concealer to neutralize the red of an occasional pimple. Use concealer to hide darkness on eyelids and under the eye. If the concealer seems too dry and shows lines, pat a tiny bit of eye cream over it. Absolutely no frosted shadows or frosted blush if you have wrinkled lids or cheeks. It's like advertising your age lines.

Magic Trick

Your eyes will look younger and fresher if you apply a light neutral shadow all over the lids first. Extremely bright eye shadow will draw attention to crepey or discolored eyelids. Medium shades or neutrals won't.

If your upper eyes are beginning to droop, sharpen the definition by lining them with a neutral (black, charcoal, or brown) powder eye shadow applied with a wet eyeliner brush. It will dry softer than liquid eyeliner but will be more defined than pencil.

When lining eyes with a pencil or powder, don't draw a thick line. It will drag the eye down. Don't line the lower lid if it's puffy, wrinkly, or dark. Curling lashes is an instant eye lift.

Mascara should be black for practically everyone, or brown if you're very fair. Colored mascara looks phony. Don't put mascara on the lower lashes when you have bags under them. If your lashes are thinning or gray, mascara is doubly important.

Perhaps you've never groomed your brows. Now's the time to start. "What's cute and fresh in your teens just looks messy when you're older," notes New York City-based makeup artist Lea Siegal. You want a natural shape—not a high fashion look. Fill in sparse brows with brow powder and the small angle brush that comes with it (Clinique has a good one). It should be charcoal or taupe—never black or brown.

If your skin seems to be losing some of its color as you age, brighten up your blush with rose for cools and coral for warms. Don't overdo. You don't want clown cheeks. Do use the facelifting application described in the makeup chapter, because it works for all ages.

If you have vertical lines around your mouth you'll want to use foundation, a special lip cream to help prevent lipstick bleeding, then follow with powder. Always line with a lip pencil. It not only helps thinning lips look larger, but the wax will help retard bleeding as well. Then try a less-vibrant shade of lipstick that won't show bleeding so easily. We've all seen the wrinkled matron with the bright red "bleeding" lipstick. If your lipstick shade is too dark it will also make your lips look smaller.

After lip liner, use your lipstick brush to apply a lipstick outline, blending lip pencil and lipstick at the same time. Finish off with the tube.

Frosted lipstick will make your lips look fuller.

Your makeup can never make you look like you had a facelift, but it can make you look healthy and rested.

 Magic Trick

If your eyes are not as good as they used to be, make an investment in a high-powered, excellent quality magnifying mirror. You'll use it every day for the rest of your life.

Tips for Brighter Teeth

As we age, our teeth discolor. Yellow teeth can add years to your age. You can have a whiter, brighter, younger smile for a relatively low price just by visiting your dentist.

Impressions are taken of your teeth and your dentist makes clear, custom plastic molds. At your second visit, the appliances are fitted and you are provided with applicators of tooth-whitening solution.

There are different methods, but one is to put the solution in the appliances and wear them at night while sleeping. After just a few nights, teeth are whiter and brighter. A follow-up application can be used every few months to maintain bright teeth.

Cosmetic Surgery

Insisting that human beings, like fine wines, get better with age sounds like sour grapes to me. Yet a good plastic surgeon can transform wrinkles into fine wine. Frown lines, smile lines, and vertical lines around the mouth can almost disappear with laser surgery.

Medical science is giving us more options every day, but do investigate thoroughly and talk to several doctors before deciding you want to have cosmetic surgery and who should do the work.

Especially facelifts. You don't want to end up looking like a dummy in a wax museum. Good cosmetic surgery should look natural and relaxed, not stiff or pulled.

Remember, hearts never get wrinkled, and that's the most important thing.

Even if you can no longer wear a micro-mini, you can always look contemporary, no matter what your age.

Ageless Fashions

Style—not age—should determine your fashion choices. There are many outfits that can span three generations perfectly.

How about a knee-length, two-piece, plain knit dress with a pleated skirt topped off with a houndstooth check tunic-length jacket? Or a silk crepe dress with long sleeves and a jewel neck? Perfect for grandmom, mom, and granddaughter. Even if you can no longer wear a micro-mini, you can always look contemporary, no matter what your age.

Hairstyle

Many women are convinced that short hair is as inevitable as menopause. (Those aren't hot flashes ladies, they are power surges.) The round shaped, extremely short style that many maturing women end up with has become a cliche for growing old. A short smart defined hairstyle is fine if it goes with the shape of your face, neck, and body. Shoulder-length hair (no longer!) and all lengths in between can look smashing on classic women, too.

Another cliche that has become a fashion joke for graying women is blue hair. That halo of blue hair says "little old lady." Blue hair rinses (like eye shadow) ought to be illegal. Instead, use a product such as Shimmer Lights by Clairol, which only shampoos away the yellow in gray or white hair without turning it blue.

Hair that is excessively long, hair that is too stiff, and especially hair that is too blond or too red or too black can add years to your image. A brassy mane of blond locks doesn't mean youth, it means tacky. It makes you look like you're trying to race back to puberty.

Magic Trick

Hair color that is roofing-tar black or traffic-cone orange spells A-G-E. Try letting your hair gray naturally, especially if you are a brunette. You will be pleasantly surprised by this elegant, classic look.

When I was in the fourth grade I had a Sunday school teacher I admired greatly. I thought she was stunning with her silver hair and high heels. Everyone else I knew then who had gray hair wore grandma shoes. This teacher was a loving and giving person to everyone in her class. I decided then that one day I would have silver hair and wear high heels. So here I am. As an added bonus, the silver "classic" look is good for my modeling. Women my age relate to me when I walk down a runway, and not to the anorexic-looking teenage model. (I also sell more clothes, because women say, "If she can look good in that outfit so can I.")

To gray or not to gray? To answer that question, ask yourself: Do I like gray hair? Does it make me feel old?

Is my gray hair pretty or mousy? During the graying process some color seasons gray attractively, some do not. Autumn and Spring will change to golden-gray, Winter and summer change to silver-gray.

Winters gray best and usually have the prettiest color. When you see gray hair that you think is striking, it's almost always someone who had dark brunette hair, a Winter person.

If you have dark brunette hair and reject the idea of going gray, be sure you see a professional hairstylist for advice. Choose a color at least two shades lighter than your original color. Hair that is too dark makes wrinkles turn on like neon lights. A flat matte color says, "I did this at home." Hair isn't all one color. Hairstylists can mix colors to give hair a natural shiny appearance.

Autumns look good when they have finished the graying cycle, but should have help from a hairdresser until they get there, semi-permanent tints, for example.

Springs should stay blond or highlight forever.

Summers are prime candidates for highlighting or weaving, as they frequently have mousy brown hair. Highlighting also works well to blend in with gray hair. It is easier to maintain because the roots can show and still look good. If allowing your hair to gray is not your thing, then try some reverse streaking. The dark streaks will mellow the grayness. Just be careful in selecting your hairstylist. He or she must know what color season you are and what is the right color shading for your hair. For instance, beige blond for Summers, golden blond for Springs.

We look different at different ages, and every age speaks for itself.

Get used to the idea of being a classic woman. As such, your face and body type will transcend trends. You will have achieved your own individual style. You are always up to date, so you don't have to follow the latest fad.

We are women. We look different at different ages, and every age speaks for itself. A woman on the forty-plus side has something to say. She is a picture that lights up. She is a woman who is fabulous at any age. As Ashleigh Brilliant, creator of "Pot Shots," said, "You can only be young once, but you can be beautiful over and over."

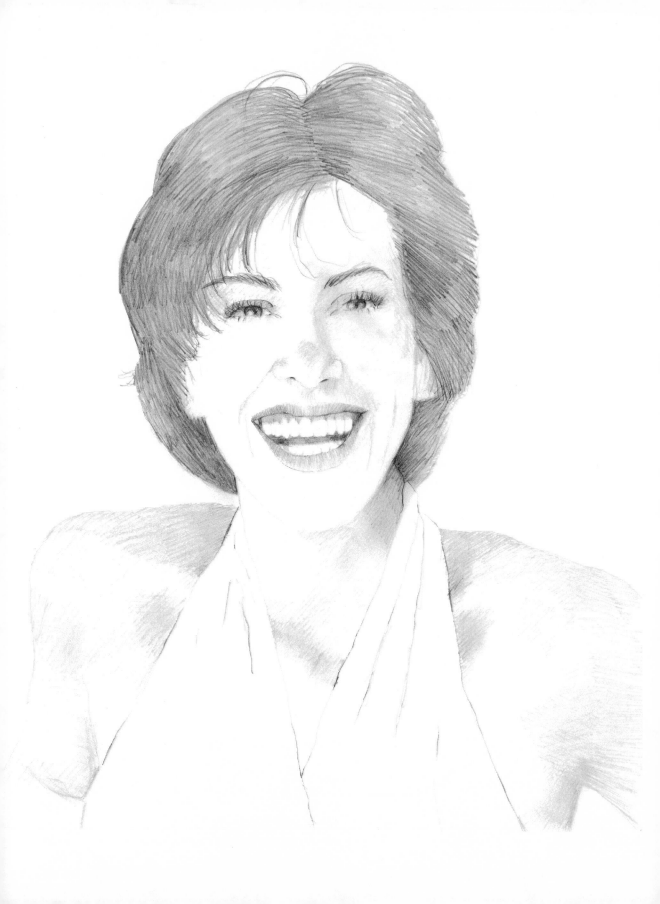

Looking Great!

For Every Woman Who Has a Body

"At a certain point in my early life, I decided what sort of person I wanted to be, and over the years I've become that person. Now I no longer remember what part of me is original and what part of me is the person I've invented. The two have merged."

—Cary Grant

Well, you've done it. You've created the "new you"—like magic.

You have used image, silhouette, lifestyle, and fashion techniques that slim and trim and enhance your special body needs.

You have improved your overall appearance through the magic of illusion by emphasizing your assets and camouflaging your faults. You have gone from so-so to so-stunning.

You are looking great!

put hands in back to fix posture
sit on edge of chair + push back
To take off jacket slide off shoulders then off arms
Picture stance stand at 12 + 10 or 12 + 2
stairs - walk whole foot on face away from rail
Black any time w/ color necklace / earrings
weekenders clothes
chico Store near Nordstrom
belts always slightly carried
Jessica's Consignment

People Love Hats

Use personal Shopper - Nordstrom (alterations free)
Pearl choker
Push up long sleeves
straight leg pants only from hips or bell
angels look thinner
get washable always
fewer pieces better quality
V neck great
metal + lace seen first
dark stockings
Purse - hand around bottom of bag